TOP 100
taste.com.AU

# THE eat REAL DIET

## YOUR ULTIMATE VEG-LOVERS' SUPER NATURAL COOKBOOK AND EATING PLAN

HarperCollins*Publishers*

# CONTENTS

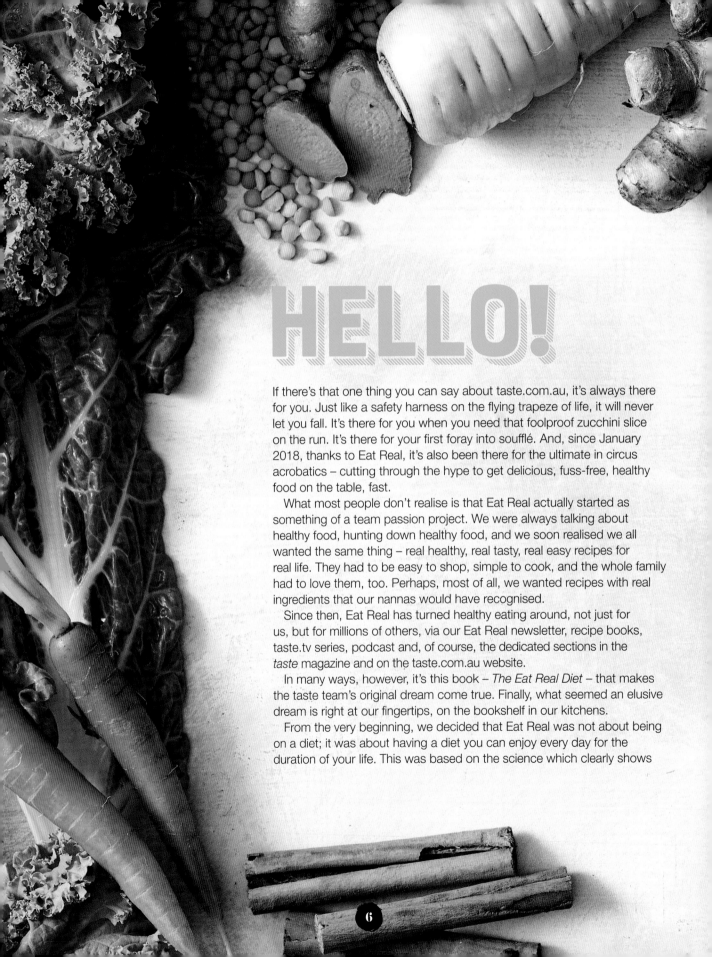

# HELLO!

If there's that one thing you can say about taste.com.au, it's always there for you. Just like a safety harness on the flying trapeze of life, it will never let you fall. It's there for you when you need that foolproof zucchini slice on the run. It's there for your first foray into soufflé. And, since January 2018, thanks to Eat Real, it's also been there for the ultimate in circus acrobatics – cutting through the hype to get delicious, fuss-free, healthy food on the table, fast.

What most people don't realise is that Eat Real actually started as something of a team passion project. We were always talking about healthy food, hunting down healthy food, and we soon realised we all wanted the same thing – real healthy, real tasty, real easy recipes for real life. They had to be easy to shop, simple to cook, and the whole family had to love them, too. Perhaps, most of all, we wanted recipes with real ingredients that our nannas would have recognised.

Since then, Eat Real has turned healthy eating around, not just for us, but for millions of others, via our Eat Real newsletter, recipe books, taste.tv series, podcast and, of course, the dedicated sections in the *taste* magazine and on the taste.com.au website.

In many ways, however, it's this book – *The Eat Real Diet* – that makes the taste team's original dream come true. Finally, what seemed an elusive dream is right at our fingertips, on the bookshelf in our kitchens.

From the very beginning, we decided that Eat Real was not about being on a diet; it was about having a diet you can enjoy every day for the duration of your life. This was based on the science which clearly shows

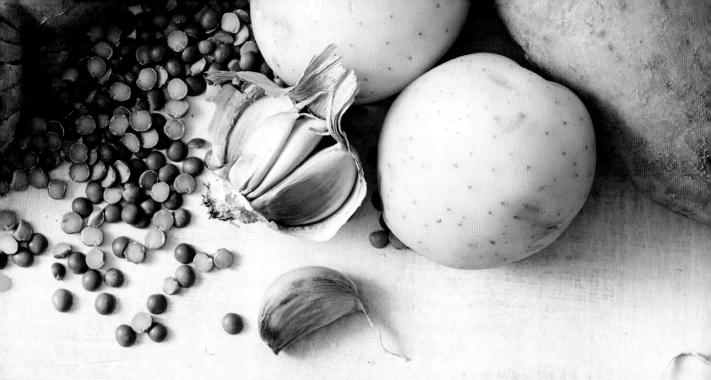

that the healthy diet you stick to really can influence both the length and quality of your life in a profound way.

With *The Eat Real Diet*, everything is designed to make healthy eating as easy as it can be. These are the recipes you want to eat as your very first preference, not the ones you 'should' eat. And, even though it's not about losing weight, you certainly have all the information you need to track calories when you want to cut those pesky kilos. Every recipe has been calorie counted for you and we've also included easy meal plans on page 29, so you can organise how you want to eat ahead of time.

If you like features, we've got features. There's a whole haul to plunder here. Check them out, from page 8. The one I know I'll use constantly is the Mix & Match guide (page 23). I can already visualise the dog ears on these pages! With handy thumbnail pics of Light Meals, Main Meals and Snacks, at-a-glance calories, and loads of useful category icons, my healthy meal planning just took a great leap forward.

And, here's another thing that makes *The Eat Real Diet* different. Whereas Eat Real, in general, takes a 'flexitarian' approach, all the recipes in this book are vegetarian or vegan – as a bonus, loads are gluten-free, too! Again, we based this on the science, backed up by our interviews and research for the Eat Real Unwrapped podcast series. As every world-leading authority we spoke to for the podcast told us, the number one thing every expert agrees on is this: eat a plant-based diet.

So, veg lovers rejoice! That singular all-in-one cookbook and meal planner you can turn to every day is all yours. Harnesses on. Let's get flying!

*Brodee*

**BRODEE MYERS,
EDITOR-IN-CHIEF**

## JOIN OUR EAT REAL COMMUNITY

◉ **EAT REAL ON TASTE.COM.AU**
taste.com.au/healthy

◉ **EAT REAL FACEBOOK PAGE**
facebook.com/tasteeatreal

◉ **EAT REAL FACEBOOK GROUP**
facebook.com/tasteeatreal/groups

◉ **EAT REAL UNWRAPPED PODCAST**
taste.com.au/eatreal/podcast

◉ **EAT REAL MONTHLY NEWSLETTER**
taste.com.au/eatreal/newsletter

To access all our Eat Real resources, scan the QR code, below.

# HOW TO USE

# THE EAT REAL DIET

Welcome to taste.com.au's *The Eat Real Diet*, with all the recipes, tools, tips and guides you need to achieve your everyday health and wellbeing goals.

# AMAZING FEATURES

Full prep & cooking times

Complete nutritional information

5-star recipe ratings

At-a-glance calorie counter

Reviews from home cooks

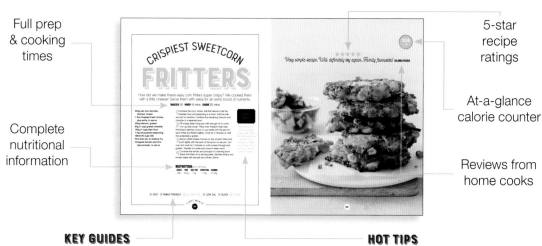

**KEY GUIDES**
Highlighted dots indicating Easy, Family-Friendly Gluten-Free, Low-Cal and Vegan meals

**HOT TIPS**
Helpful hints, including easy swaps, make-ahead advice and nutrition know-how

# DO IT YOUR WAY

All our recipes are divided into three main sections: Light Meals, Main Meals and Snacks. Plus, we've done the calorie counting for you, so you don't have to!

## LIGHT MEALS
### UP TO 400 CALORIES

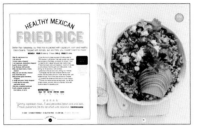

Turn here for breakfast, lunch and lighter dinner ideas, while keeping your calorie intake on track, page 31.

## MAIN MEALS
### UP TO 600 CALORIES

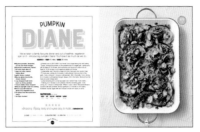

Hearty yet healthy, our main meals are stacked with your favourite plant-based ingredients, page 123.

## SNACKS
### UP TO 250 CALORIES

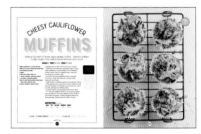

We've got all your healthy bases covered for when a snack-attack strikes. You're spoilt for choice, page 215.

# MIX & MATCH GUIDES

Here's your daily and weekly meal planner where you can see every meal at a glance, with key guides, calorie count and page number listed on each recipe.

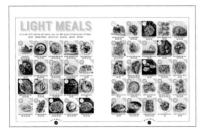

You can plan your days simply and quickly by choosing your favourite lighter meal options that are low-cal, delicious and filling, page 24.

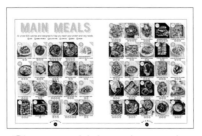

Choose which mains you're having based on calories and dietary requirements. They're all designed to help you reach your protein and veg needs, page 26.

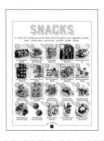

Did someone say snacks? Prevent hunger, satisfy any cravings and supplement your wellbeing with these tasty snack options, page 28.

# INDEXES

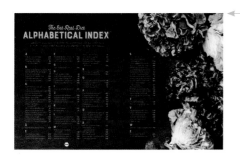

## INDEX BY ALPHBETICAL

Know what you're looking for? Find it easily in our handy alphabetical guide, page 246.

## INDEX BY KEY GUIDE

This index sorts the recipes according to special criteria, such as Easy, Family-Friendly Gluten-Free, Low-Cal and Vegan. Satisfy everyone, page 248.

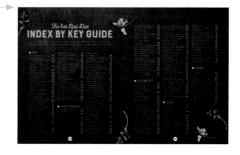

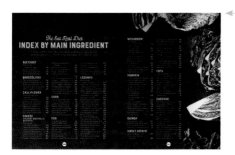

## INDEX BY MAIN INGREDIENT

This quick finder helps you locate all your main protein and vegetable options, so that you can eat what you love, plus increase the overall nutrients in your diet, page 250.

## INDEX BY MEAL TYPE

We've listed all the meals under Light meals, Main meals and Snacks, so you can jump straight to your heart's desire, page 252.

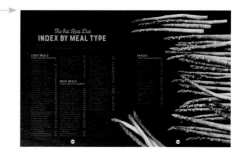

# HANDY GUIDES

To help keep you on track with your healthy eating goals,
we've included a wealth of other handy features in *The Eat Real Diet*.

## EASY MEAL PLANS

Here's your formula for building your daily meal plans, based on our pre-calculated calories. Take a look at our sample plans, then choose your meals from the Mix & Match guides. Or create your own daily plans and targets – everything you need to customise *The Eat Real Diet* is at your fingertips, page 29.

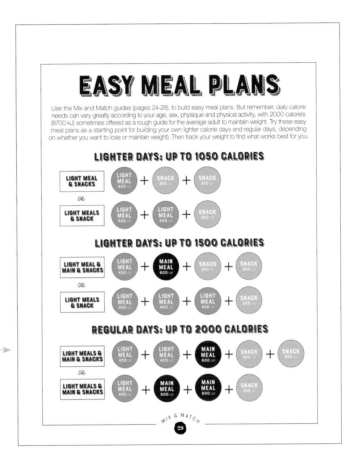

### EASY MEAL PLANS

Use the Mix and Match guides (pages 24-28), to build easy meal plans. But remember, daily calorie needs can vary greatly according to your age, sex, physique and physical activity, with 2000 calories (8700 kJ) sometimes offered as a rough guide for the average adult to maintain weight. Try these easy meal plans as a starting point for building your own lighter calorie days and regular days, depending on whether you want to lose or maintain weight. Then track your weight to find what works best for you.

**LIGHTER DAYS: UP TO 1050 CALORIES**

LIGHT MEAL & SNACKS: LIGHT MEAL 400 cal + SNACK 250 cal + SNACK 250 cal

*or*

LIGHT MEALS & SNACK: LIGHT MEAL 400 cal + LIGHT MEAL 400 cal + SNACK 250 cal

**LIGHTER DAYS: UP TO 1500 CALORIES**

LIGHT MEAL & MAIN & SNACKS: LIGHT MEAL 400 cal + MAIN MEAL 600 cal + SNACK 250 cal + SNACK 250 cal

*or*

LIGHT MEALS & SNACK: LIGHT MEAL 400 cal + LIGHT MEAL 400 cal + LIGHT MEAL 400 cal + SNACK 250 cal

**REGULAR DAYS: UP TO 2000 CALORIES**

LIGHT MEALS & MAIN & SNACKS: LIGHT MEAL 400 cal + LIGHT MEAL 400 cal + MAIN MEAL 600 cal + SNACK 250 cal + SNACK 250 cal

*or*

LIGHT MEALS & MAIN & SNACKS: LIGHT MEAL 400 cal + MAIN MEAL 600 cal + MAIN MEAL 600 cal + SNACK 250 cal

MIX & MATCH
**29**

## THE TASTE.COM.AU GUARANTEE

All taste.com.au recipes are triple-tested, rated and reviewed by Aussie cooks just like you. Plus, every ingredient is as close as your local supermarket.

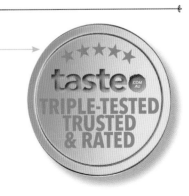

taste.com.au
TRIPLE-TESTED
TRUSTED
& RATED

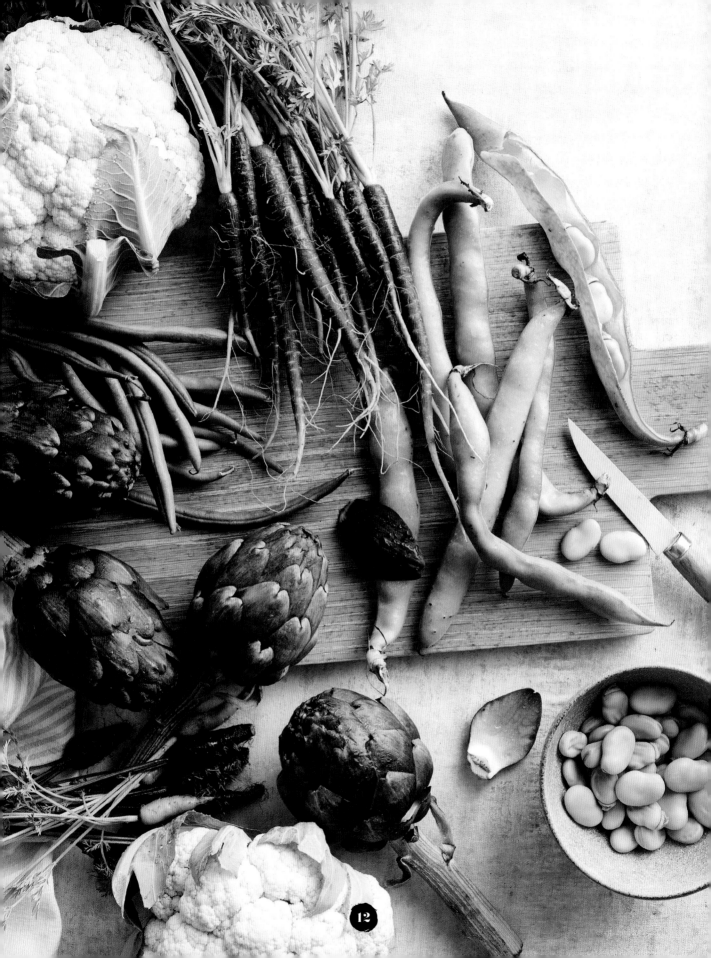

# ALL ABOUT *eat* REAL

At taste, we want to help you get real about healthy eating. Eating healthy food does *not* mean you have to jump onto a diet fad, spend lots of time and money on ingredients and eat dishes that taste like cardboard. Eat Real makes healthy eating simple, achievable and super tasty. It's all about enjoyment and balance. In fact, no favourite foods are completely off the menu. There's even room for treats and the odd glass of wine! We're talking real food, with real taste that's real healthy. So, let's get real together!

Welcome to taste.com.au's Eat Real. Before we get into the nitty gritty, you need to know that Eat Real is not about being 'on a diet'. But you might lose a kilo or two, just because you're eating healthier foods.

We understand that eating well shouldn't feel like a chore, and it shouldn't be about sacrificing all the enjoyment you get from food (only to slip back into old eating patterns again). Eating Real is about making small changes every day to help you hit your health goals; the kind of easy changes that can make all the difference and last a lifetime.

Eat Real is about having lots of healthy food ideas and choices at your fingertips, with thousands of recipes to suit every person, every family, taste preferences and special dietary requirements, such as gluten free and vegan. Never before has eating healthier food been so incredibly easy for everyone!

## REAL HEALTHY

Have you been struggling to meet your healthy eating goals? With so many health myths, impossible diet rules and everyday-life hurdles, it's not easy to cut through to what's real about healthy eating.

We're setting the record straight on health fads, confusing diet trends and impractical food rules. Why? Because you shouldn't have to starve yourself or spend your days tallying up calories and grams of fat for every bit of food that touches your lips. We're here to show you that healthy eating isn't complicated; it's simply about making good choices.

## REAL LIFE

We totally understand that eating healthy is not 'one size fits all', so Eat Real will help you wherever you're at on your path to healthy. You can bring your family along, too – they'll love our healthier versions of favourite dinners.

Every dietary need and preference is covered, so even the fussiest of eaters will find something they like.

You can dip in and out of our healthier recipes as you like, or go all the way with our pre-calorie-counted and nutritionally balanced recipes and snacks.

## REAL QUICK & EASY

Eat Real is hassle-free all the way. Many recipes are quick, easy, or can be prepped ahead. We've even done all the calorie counting for you, plus separated the meals into light meals, main meals and snacks, so that you can spend more time enjoying the food rather than agonising over it. Eat Real is your new everyday 'go-to' for any meal and every occasion, including entertaining.

## REAL BUDGET

We're all watching our bank account, and Eat Real is in tune with keeping your weekly food bills down. Eat Real ingredients are easily found in your local supermarket, so you may just find you're saving money, especially when you're using our handy online shopping tools and meal-planning guides.

## REAL STORIES

Eat Real is becoming a vibrant community, all about sharing tips, lessons learned and clever ideas. We look forward to hearing about your experiences, too – what works (and what doesn't), along with those small game-changing gems that can make a difference for someone else. We're all in this together – the whole taste.com.au community. And there's no time like the present to begin eating real!

*Eat Real is not about being 'on a diet'. But you might lose a kilo or two just because you're eating healthier foods.*

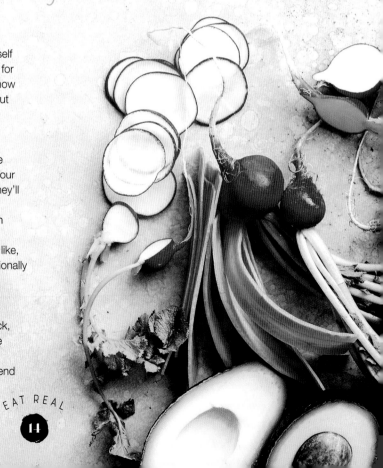

EAT REAL

# EAT REAL YOUR WAY!

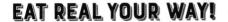

- ● Choice – you can dive into plant-based eating full time or simply increase your intake of vegetables by adding a few more vegie meals to your diet.
- ● Themes – bring your family along and plan 'meat-free Mondays' or turn 'taco Tuesdays' veg only.
- ● Twist it – add a side of chicken, seafood or meat to our plant-based recipes for a more flexitarian approach, or make simple swaps like using plant-based instead of dairy options to make a recipe work for your dietary requirements.
- ● Goals – use our meal planners and eat lighter, veg-based meals for a set period to trim down for summer or a special event.

# VEG POWER

RAMP UP THE VEGIES IN YOUR EVERYDAY EATING
TO BOOST YOUR HEALTH AND HAPPINESS.

# SUPER NATURAL POWERS

One of the key innovations introduced for *The Eat Real Diet* is an emphasis on recipes that hero vegetables. This is based on the latest science which points to the enormous role vegetables play in both health and happiness.

## WHY WE ALL NEED VEGETABLES

Health experts now consider vegetables the most important food group. In fact, unlike any other food group, we are free to eat unlimited serves!

No other food group provides so many nutrients for such little calorie content. Think of vegetables as the ultimate wholefoods, with no preservatives, additives, salts, fats or artificial sugars. Aside from the obvious nutrition benefits, with two out of three Australians overweight or obese, increasing our vegie intake can be one of the easiest and most effective ways of achieving and maintaining a healthy weight.

All vegies are healthy, however the brassica family shines with stars such as cabbage, broccoli, cauliflower, dark leafy greens and Asian greens. They are jam-packed with vitamins A, C and K, dietary fibre as well as disease-fighting phytonutrients which can keep your heart healthy and certain cancers at bay.

As for fruit, moderation is key. While it's good for you, too – think vitamin C, B vitamins, betacarotene, potassium, antioxidants and dietary fibre – fruit is high in natural sugars (fructose), so can really pile on the calories, if you're not careful. The trick is to choose fresh fruit over dried fruit and store-bought juices. Berries are great, as they are quite low in sugar and packed with antioxidants. Meanwhile, citrus provides a hefty dose of vitamin C, and fruit with edible skin, such as apples or pears, offers the most dietary fibre.

## EATING VEGIES MAKES YOU HAPPY

Scientists have also proven that as well as keeping you healthy and preventing disease, eating more fruit and veg can boost your happiness levels.

The recent study by researchers from the University of Warwick in the UK and the University of Queensland found that people who went from eating virtually no fruit and veg to eating eight portions of fruit and veg each day experienced an increase in life satisfaction equivalent to moving from unemployment to employment. And that's before they even started to reap all the physical health benefits!

Given that eating a rainbow of fruit and veg can lead to a rainbow of happiness, it's interesting that the National Health Survey discovered that only around one in 20 of us are meeting both daily quotas. This means that most Australian adults are still not having the recommended five or more serves of vegetables and two or more serves of fruit each day.

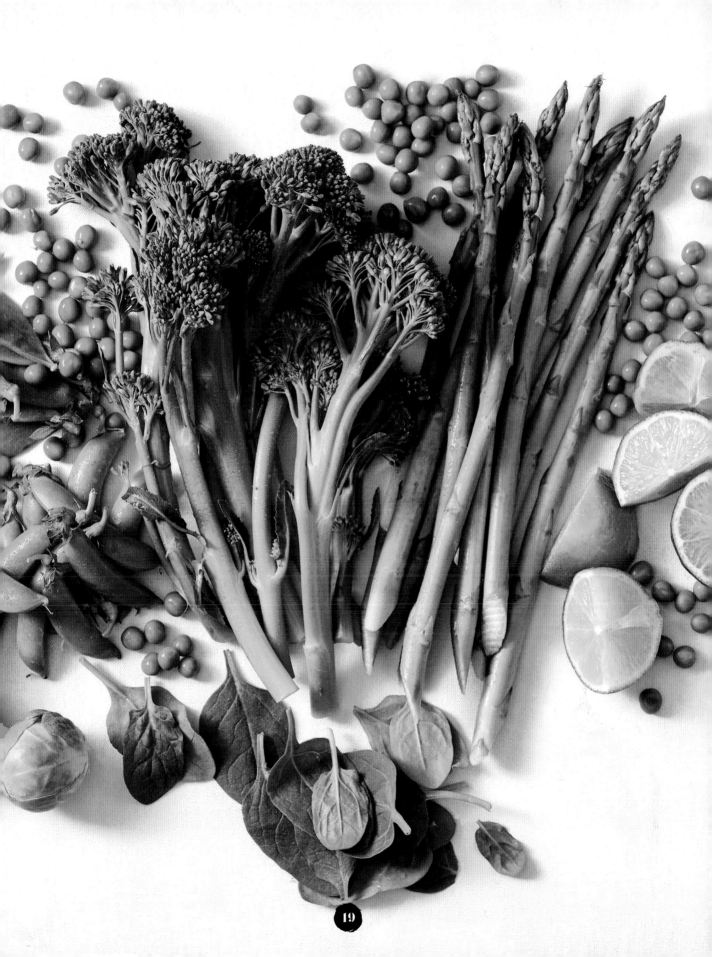

# YOUR GUIDE TO SERVINGS

Whether you are vegetarian, vegan or into plant-based eating with a little meat or seafood on the side, everyone needs to eat five serves of vegetables and two serves of fruit each day in order to meet their nutrient requirements. Variety is key. Every fruit and veg has its own vital mix of vitamins, minerals and antioxidants. To ensure your protein needs are covered, all recipes in *The Eat Real Diet* tick the box for protein, thanks to the inclusion of key plant nutrients such as nuts, seeds, legumes, beans, whole grains, tofu and tempeh.

## HOW MUCH IS A SERVE?

### VEGETABLES
#### 5+ SERVES A DAY

ONE SERVE = 75g

**TRY THESE**
- ½ cup dense vegetables (e.g. beans, corn kernels, peas)
- ½ cup cooked dried or canned legumes (e.g. lentils, chickpeas, beans)
- 1 cup green leafy or raw salad vegetables
- ½ medium potato or sweet potato
- 1 medium tomato

**ACTION PLAN**
- Eat a veg from each colour (red, green, orange, white) per day.
- Add a large handful of spinach to your morning smoothie.
- Keep raw vegie sticks on hand for a healthy snack with hummus, or turn to our Snacks (page 215).
- Steam extra veg at dinner to throw into salads for lunch the next day.

### FRUIT
#### 2+ SERVES A DAY

ONE SERVE = 150g

**TRY THESE**
- 1 medium-sized piece of fruit (le.g. apple, banana, orange or pear)
- 2 smaller fruits (e.g. apricot, kiwifruit, plum)
- 1 cup canned (no added sugar) or chopped fresh fruit (e.g. melon, pineapple)
- ½ cup (125ml) 100% fruit juice
- 1½ tbs dried fruit (e.g. sultanas or 4 dried apricot halves)

**ACTION PLAN**
- Make a fruit smoothie with frozen berries and banana for a quick and easy breakfast or snack.
- Reach for fruit containing fibre (like a green apple) as a snack when you hit the 3pm slump.
- If eating canned fruit, always choose natural products or those in water to avoid added sugars.
- More is not always better – keep total fruit serves to less than four a day, to prevent your blood sugar levels spiking.

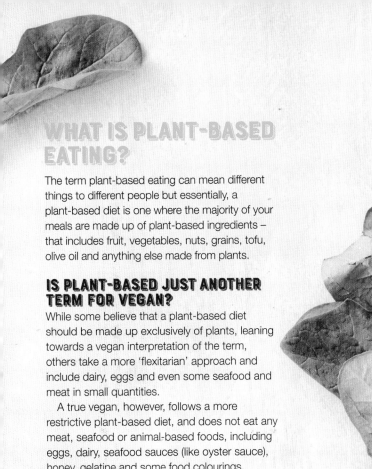

# WHAT IS PLANT-BASED EATING?

The term plant-based eating can mean different things to different people but essentially, a plant-based diet is one where the majority of your meals are made up of plant-based ingredients – that includes fruit, vegetables, nuts, grains, tofu, olive oil and anything else made from plants.

## IS PLANT-BASED JUST ANOTHER TERM FOR VEGAN?

While some believe that a plant-based diet should be made up exclusively of plants, leaning towards a vegan interpretation of the term, others take a more 'flexitarian' approach and include dairy, eggs and even some seafood and meat in small quantities.

A true vegan, however, follows a more restrictive plant-based diet, and does not eat any meat, seafood or animal-based foods, including eggs, dairy, seafood sauces (like oyster sauce), honey, gelatine and some food colourings.

## WHAT ABOUT VEGETARIANS?

Vegetarians are based firmly in the plant-based camp, with plants making up the main portion of their daily eating plan. Similar to vegans, vegetarians do not eat meat, poultry or seafood. The main difference between a vegan and those who identify themselves as a more 'traditional' vegetarian (known as lacto-ovo vegetarian), is that a lacto-ovo vegetarian will include dairy and eggs in their day-to-day diet.

The majority of recipes in this book are based on the lacto-ovo style of vegetarian eating, so they feature eggs and dairy. But don't despair if you're vegan, you'll find a decent amount of recipes and ideas for you to enjoy too – simply look out for the 'vegan' tag on the recipe, or turn to page 249 for a full list.

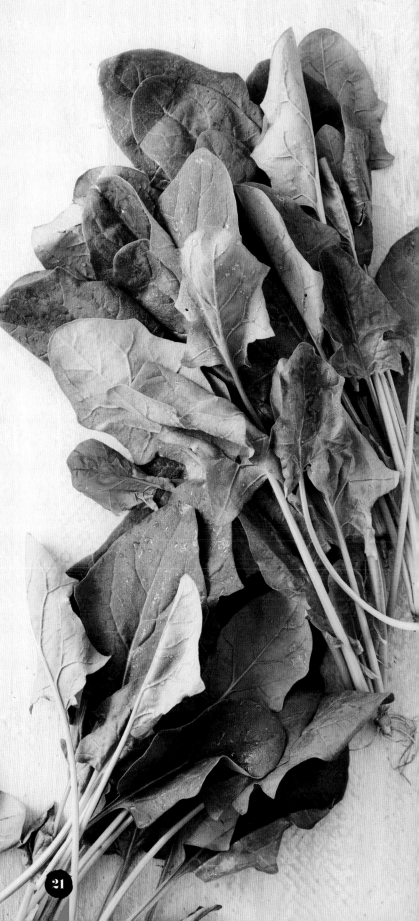

# MIX & MATCH

THIS AT-A-GLANCE GUIDE WILL MAKE IT EASY TO
PLAN YOUR FULFILLING LOW-CAL MENU EACH DAY.

# LIGHT MEALS

At under 400 calories per serve, you can feel good choosing any of these.

**E** EASY  **FF** FAMILY-FRIENDLY  **GF** GLUTEN FREE  **LC** LOW-CAL  **Q** QUICK  **V** VEGAN

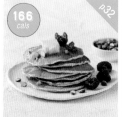
166 cals — p32
**KETO PANCAKES**
E GF LC Q

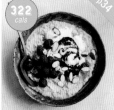
322 cals — p34
**OVERNIGHT CHIA PORRIDGE**
E LC V

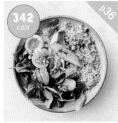
342 cals — p36
**PUNCHY PROTEIN BREAKFAST BOWL**
E GF LC Q

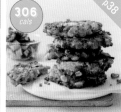
306 cals — p38
**CRISPIEST SWEETCORN FRITTERS**
E FF LC Q

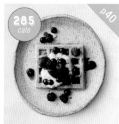
285 cals — p40
**HEALTHY BANANA WAFFLES**
E FF LC Q

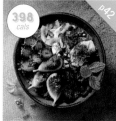
398 cals — p42
**CHOC, FRUIT & OAT BREKKY BOWL**
FF LC

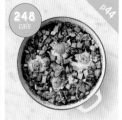
248 cals — p44
**ONE-PAN SWEET POTATO & EGG HASH**
E GF LC

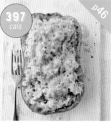
397 cals — p46
**PUMPKIN & BASIL RISOTTO**
E FF GF LC

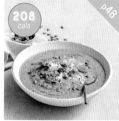
208 cals — p48
**HEALTHY LEEK & BROCCOLI SOUP**
E FF LC

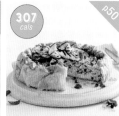
307 cals — p50
**ZUCCHINI & HALOUMI QUICHE**
FF LC

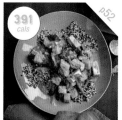
391 cals — p52
**PUMPKIN CURRY WITH TOFU**
GF LC V

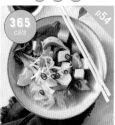
365 cals — p54
**'VEGTASTIC' PHO**
GF LC V

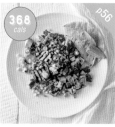
368 cals — p56
**TOFU, CORN & MUNG BEAN SALSA**
GF LC V

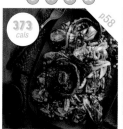
373 cals — p58
**LENTIL, BRUSSELS & MUSHIE MEDLEY**
GF LC

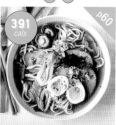
391 cals — p60
**VEGETARIAN RAMEN BOWL**
LC

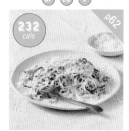
232 cals — p62
**ONE-POT KETO ZUCCHINI ALFREDO**
E GF LC Q

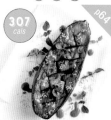
307 cals — p64
**MISO ROASTED EGGPLANT**
E GF LC

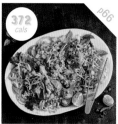
372 cals — p66
**QUICK THAI TOFU NOODLE SALAD**
GF LC Q V

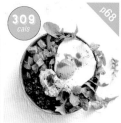
309 cals — p68
**SPICY TOMATO BLACK BEAN BOWL**
E FF GF LC

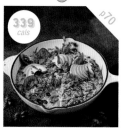
339 cals — p70
**MEXICAN ZUCCHINI SLICE**
FF LC Q

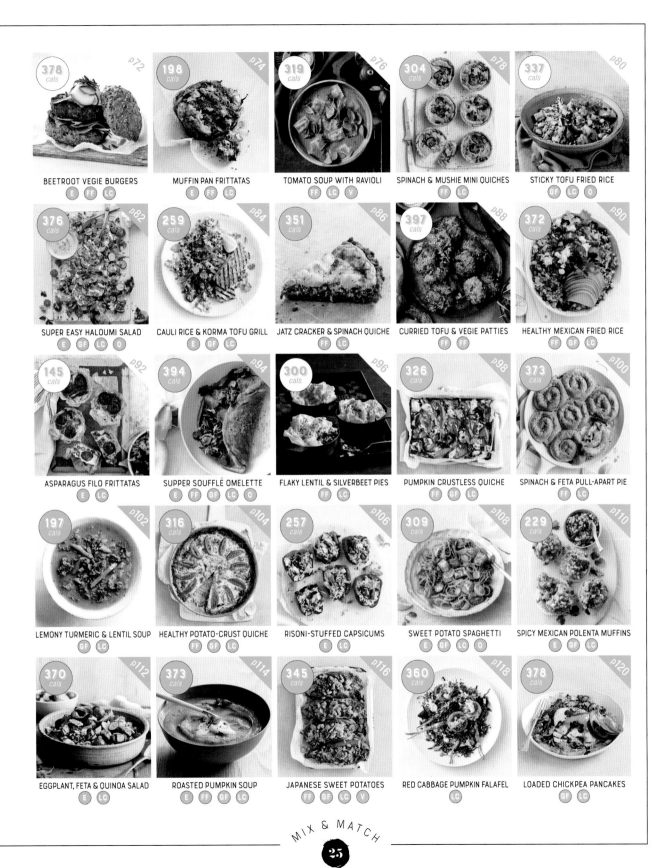

**378** cals — p72 — BEETROOT VEGIE BURGERS — E FF LC

**198** cals — p74 — MUFFIN PAN FRITTATAS — E FF LC

**319** cals — p76 — TOMATO SOUP WITH RAVIOLI — FF LC V

**304** cals — p78 — SPINACH & MUSHIE MINI QUICHES — FF LC

**337** cals — p80 — STICKY TOFU FRIED RICE — GF LC Q

**376** cals — p82 — SUPER EASY HALOUMI SALAD — E GF LC Q

**259** cals — p84 — CAULI RICE & KORMA TOFU GRILL — E GF LC

**351** cals — p86 — JATZ CRACKER & SPINACH QUICHE — E GF LC

**397** cals — p88 — CURRIED TOFU & VEGIE PATTIES — FF LC

**372** cals — p90 — HEALTHY MEXICAN FRIED RICE — E GF LC

**145** cals — p92 — ASPARAGUS FILO FRITTATAS — E LC

**394** cals — p94 — SUPPER SOUFFLÉ OMELETTE — E FF GF LC Q

**300** cals — p96 — FLAKY LENTIL & SILVERBEET PIES — FF LC

**326** cals — p98 — PUMPKIN CRUSTLESS QUICHE — FF GF LC

**373** cals — p100 — SPINACH & FETA PULL-APART PIE — FF LC

**197** cals — p102 — LEMONY TURMERIC & LENTIL SOUP — GF LC

**316** cals — p104 — HEALTHY POTATO-CRUST QUICHE — FF GF LC

**257** cals — p106 — RISONI-STUFFED CAPSICUMS — E LC

**309** cals — p108 — SWEET POTATO SPAGHETTI — E GF LC Q

**229** cals — p110 — SPICY MEXICAN POLENTA MUFFINS — E GF LC

**370** cals — p112 — EGGPLANT, FETA & QUINOA SALAD — E LC

**373** cals — p114 — ROASTED PUMPKIN SOUP — E FF GF LC

**345** cals — p116 — JAPANESE SWEET POTATOES — FF GF LC V

**360** cals — p118 — RED CABBAGE PUMPKIN FALAFEL — LC

**378** cals — p120 — LOADED CHICKPEA PANCAKES — GF LC

# MAIN MEALS

All under 600 calories and designed to help you reach your protein and veg needs.

**E** EASY  **FF** FAMILY-FRIENDLY  **GF** GLUTEN FREE  **LC** LOW-CAL  **Q** QUICK  **V** VEGAN

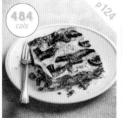
p124 · 484 cals

**MUSHROOM & LENTIL LASAGNE**
FF LC

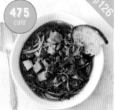
p126 · 475 cals

**QUICK VEGETARIAN MINESTRONE**
E FF LC

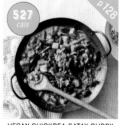
p128 · 527 cals

**VEGAN CHICKPEA SATAY CURRY**
E FF LC Q V

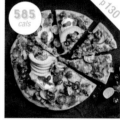
p130 · 585 cals

**MEXICAN TACO PIZZAS**
E FF LC Q

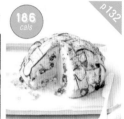
p132 · 186 cals

**CHEESY-STUFFED CAULIFLOWER**
LC

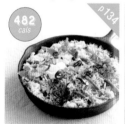
p134 · 482 cals

**ONE-PAN VEGETABLE BIRYANI**
E FF LC

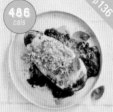
p136 · 486 cals

**EGGPLANT PARMIGIANA**
E FF LC

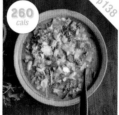
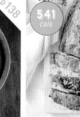
p138 · 260 cals

**HEALTHY TUSCAN BREAD SOUP**
E LC

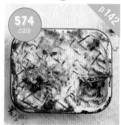
p140 · 541 cals

**VEGETABLE WELLINGTON**
FF LC

p142 · 574 cals

**LASAGNE WITH ZUCCHINI LATTICE**
FF LC

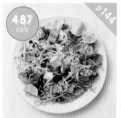
p144 · 487 cals

**QUICK VEGETARIAN PAD THAI**
E LC Q

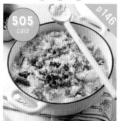
p146 · 505 cals

**RISOTTO PRIMAVERA**
FF LC

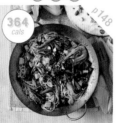
p148 · 364 cals

**QUICK SUPER-GREEN MEE GORENG**
E FF LC Q

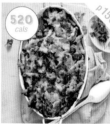
p150 · 520 cals

**MUSHROOM STROGANOFF BAKE**
E FF LC

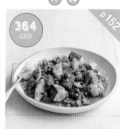
p152 · 364 cals

**NORTH INDIAN PANEER CURRY**
GF LC

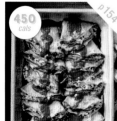
p154 · 450 cals

**STUFFED BUCKWHEAT CRESPELLE**
FF GF LC

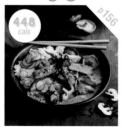
p156 · 448 cals

**JAPANESE TOFU KATSU**
LC

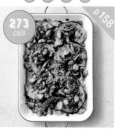
p158 · 273 cals

**PUMPKIN DIANE**
E GF LC

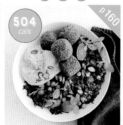
p160 · 504 cals

**FALAFEL & BLACK RICE TABOULI**
E GF LC Q V

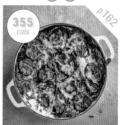
p162 · 355 cals

**EGGPLANT PARMIGIANA LASAGNE**
FF LC

MIX & MATCH

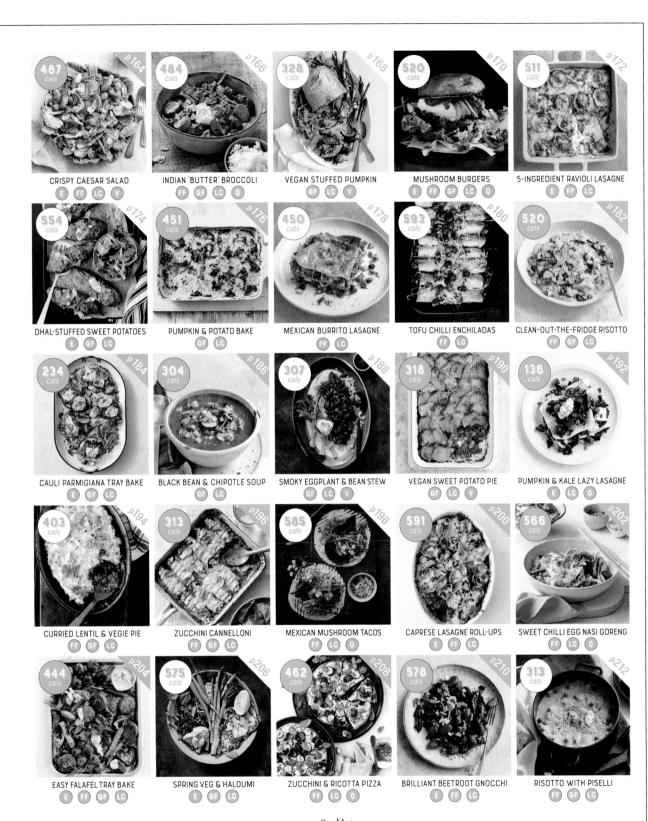

**487** cals — p164 — CRISPY CAESAR SALAD — E FF LC V

**484** cals — p166 — INDIAN 'BUTTER' BROCCOLI — FF GF LC Q

**328** cals — p168 — VEGAN STUFFED PUMPKIN — GF LC V

**520** cals — p170 — MUSHROOM BURGERS — E FF GF LC Q

**511** cals — p172 — 5-INGREDIENT RAVIOLI LASAGNE — E FF LC

**554** cals — p174 — DHAL-STUFFED SWEET POTATOES — E GF LC

**451** cals — p176 — PUMPKIN & POTATO BAKE — GF LC

**450** cals — p178 — MEXICAN BURRITO LASAGNE — FF LC

**593** cals — p180 — TOFU CHILLI ENCHILADAS — FF LC

**520** cals — p182 — CLEAN-OUT-THE-FRIDGE RISOTTO — FF GF LC

**234** cals — p184 — CAULI PARMIGIANA TRAY BAKE — E GF LC

**304** cals — p186 — BLACK BEAN & CHIPOTLE SOUP — GF LC

**307** cals — p188 — SMOKY EGGPLANT & BEAN STEW — GF LC V

**318** cals — p190 — VEGAN SWEET POTATO PIE — GF LC V

**136** cals — p192 — PUMPKIN & KALE LAZY LASAGNE — E LC Q

**403** cals — p194 — CURRIED LENTIL & VEGIE PIE — FF GF LC

**313** cals — p196 — ZUCCHINI CANNELLONI — FF GF LC

**585** cals — p198 — MEXICAN MUSHROOM TACOS — FF LC Q

**591** cals — p200 — CAPRESE LASAGNE ROLL-UPS — E FF LC

**566** cals — p202 — SWEET CHILLI EGG NASI GORENG — FF LC Q

**444** cals — p204 — EASY FALAFEL TRAY BAKE — E FF GF LC

**575** cals — p206 — SPRING VEG & HALOUMI — E GF LC

**462** cals — p208 — ZUCCHINI & RICOTTA PIZZA — FF LC Q

**578** cals — p210 — BRILLIANT BEETROOT GNOCCHI — E FF LC

**313** cals — p212 — RISOTTO WITH PISELLI — FF GF LC

# SNACKS

At under 250 calories per serve, these will fill the gaps in your appetite guilt-free.

**E** EASY    **FF** FAMILY-FRIENDLY    **GF** GLUTEN FREE    **LC** LOW-CAL    **Q** QUICK    **V** VEGAN

**200** cals — p216
**GARLIC BREAD DOUGHNUTS**
FF LC

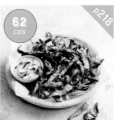

**62** cals — p218
**AIR FRYER VEGIE PEEL CRISPS**
E FF GF LC

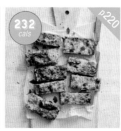

**232** cals — p220
**KETO GARLIC BREAD**
FF GF LC

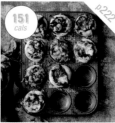

**151** cals — p222
**NICE 'N' EASY PIZZA MUFFINS**
E FF LC

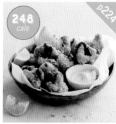

**248** cals — p224
**JAPANESE FRIED CAULIFLOWER**
LC

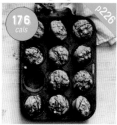

**176** cals — p226
**ZUCCHINI & FETA MUFFINS**
E FF LC

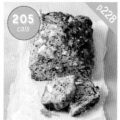

**205** cals — p228
**VEGETABLE PEEL & FETA LOAF**
E FF LC

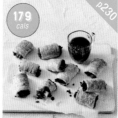

**179** cals — p230
**CHEESY VEG 'SAUSAGE' ROLLS**
FF LC

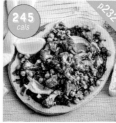

**245** cals — p232
**SPICED CAULI & HUMMUS DIP**
E LC Q

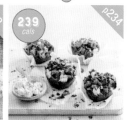

**239** cals — p234
**PUMPKIN & RICOTTA MUFFINS**
FF LC

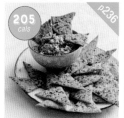

**205** cals — p236
**CHEESY KETO SNACKS**
E FF GF LC Q

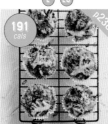

**191** cals — p238
**CHEESY CAULIFLOWER MUFFINS**
E FF LC

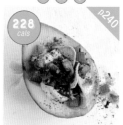

**145** cals — p240
**CARROT TOP PESTO**
E FF GF LC Q

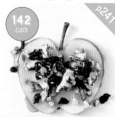

**228** cals — p240
**SALSA FUN AVOCADO**
E FF GF LC Q

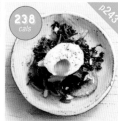

**142** cals — p241
**APPLE BRUSCHETTA SLICES**
E FF GF LC Q

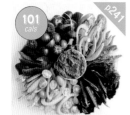

**101** cals — p241
**RAINBOW BEETROOT DRIP**
E FF GF LC Q

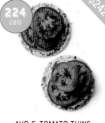

**224** cals — p242
**AVO & TOMATO THINS**
E FF GF LC Q

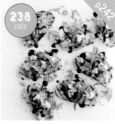

**238** cals — p242
**ROAST VEGIE TOASTIES**
E FF LC

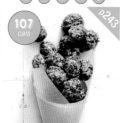

**107** cals — p243
**BROCCOLI QUINOA NUGGETS**
E FF GF LC

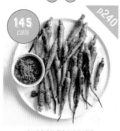

**238** cals — p243
**POACHED EGG & KALE SNACK**
E FF LC Q

# EASY MEAL PLANS

Use the Mix and Match guides (pages 24-28), to build easy meal plans. But remember, daily calorie needs can vary greatly according to your age, sex, physique and physical activity, with 2000 calories (8700 kJ) sometimes offered as a rough guide for the average adult to maintain weight. Try these easy meal plans as a starting point for building your own lighter calorie days and regular days, depending on whether you want to lose or maintain weight). Then track your weight to find what works best for you.

## LIGHTER DAYS: UP TO 1050 CALORIES

| LIGHT MEAL & SNACKS | LIGHT MEAL 400 cal | + | SNACK 250 cal | + | SNACK 250 cal |

OR

| LIGHT MEALS & SNACK | LIGHT MEAL 400 cal | + | LIGHT MEAL 400 cal | + | SNACK 250 cal |

## LIGHTER DAYS: UP TO 1500 CALORIES

| LIGHT MEAL & MAIN & SNACKS | LIGHT MEAL 400 cal | + | MAIN MEAL 600 cal | + | SNACK 250 cal | + | SNACK 250 cal |

OR

| LIGHT MEALS & SNACK | LIGHT MEAL 400 cal | + | LIGHT MEAL 400 cal | + | LIGHT MEAL 400 cal | + | SNACK 250 cal |

## REGULAR DAYS: UP TO 2000 CALORIES

| LIGHT MEALS & MAIN & SNACKS | LIGHT MEAL 400 cal | + | LIGHT MEAL 400 cal | + | MAIN MEAL 600 cal | + | SNACK 250 cal | + | SNACK 250 cal |

OR

| LIGHT MEAL & MAIN & SNACKS | LIGHT MEAL 400 cal | + | MAIN MEAL 600 cal | + | MAIN MEAL 600 cal | + | SNACK 250 cal |

# LIGHT MEALS

LOWER-CAL, FULL-OF-FLAVOUR DISHES YOU'LL LOVE.
THEY'RE ALL UNDER 400 CALORIES PER SERVE!

# KETO
# PANCAKES

Made from almond flour – high in healthy fats and fibre – cream cheese and eggs, these ketogenic diet pancakes are low carb and worth flipping over.

**MAKES** 10   **PREP** 5 mins   **COOK** 10 mins

80g (⅔ cup) almond meal
125g cream cheese, chopped,
   at room temperature
3 eggs
1 tsp vanilla extract
¼ tsp gluten-free baking powder
Butter, to cook, plus extra, to serve
Pistachios, chopped, to serve
Fresh raspberries,
   to serve (optional)

**1** Use a wooden spoon to beat the almond meal and cream cheese in a bowl until combined. Gradually beat in the eggs until well combined and lump free. Stir in the vanilla and baking powder.

**2** Working in batches, place a little butter in a non-stick frying pan over medium heat. Pour ¼ cup of batter into the pan for each pancake. Cook for 2 minutes or until undersides are golden. Carefully turn over (they will be a bit fragile) and cook for a further 1 minute. Transfer to a plate.

**3** Serve pancakes topped with extra butter, pistachio and the raspberries, if using.

**COOK'S NOTE**

If you like, cook smaller pikelet-sized pancakes to take to work or school for morning tea.

## NUTRITION (PER PANCAKE)

| CALS | FAT | SAT FAT | PROTEIN | CARBS |
|------|------|---------|---------|-------|
| 166 | 15.8g | 6.6g | 5.1g | 0.9g |

★★★★★

*So yummy. Worked out perfectly. I added a pinch of salt to the mixture. We enjoyed it with whipped cream and fresh blueberries and raspberries. Great start to the day.* **VMOXHAM**

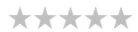 ● EASY   ○ FAMILY-FRIENDLY   ● GLUTEN FREE   ● LOW CAL   ● QUICK   ○ VEGAN

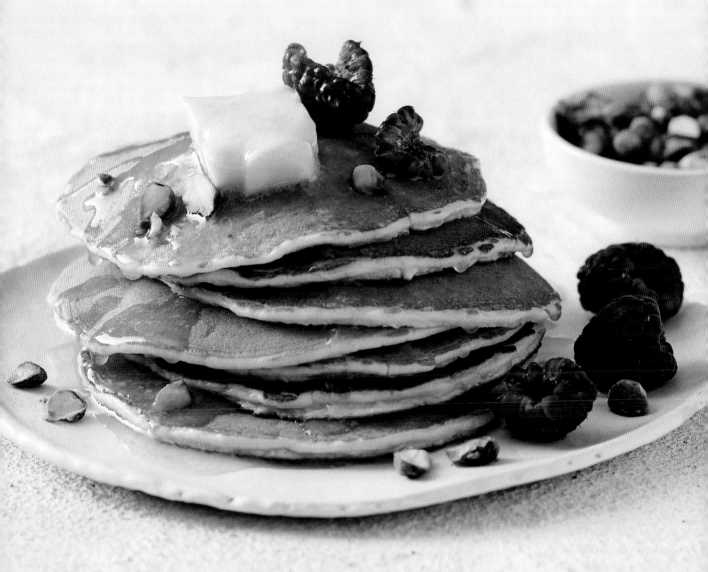

# OVERNIGHT CHIA
# PORRIDGE

Supercharge your oats and seeds while you sleep for the perfect healthy breakfast. Pimp it up with five delicious toppings, then dig in!

**SERVES** 2  **PREP** 10 mins (+ overnight soaking)  **COOK** 10 mins

50g (½ cup) traditional rolled oats
2 tbs chia seeds
¼ tsp ground cinnamon
500ml (2 cups) almond milk
Dairy-free yoghurt, to serve
Raspberry jam, to swirl
Maple syrup, to drizzle
Fresh raspberries, to serve
Natural sliced almonds, to sprinkle

1 Combine the oats, chia seeds, cinnamon and almond milk in a bowl. Cover with plastic wrap and place in the fridge to soak overnight.

2 Transfer the oat mixture to a saucepan. Cook, stirring, over medium-low heat for 5-10 minutes or until the mixture is thick and creamy.

3 Divide porridge among 2 serving bowls. Spoon yoghurt on top and swirl in some jam. Drizzle over a little maple syrup. Scatter with raspberries and almond, to serve.

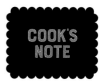

**COOK'S NOTE**

If watching your sugar intake, swap the jam for fresh fruit coulis.

## NUTRITION (PER SERVE)

| CALS | FAT | SAT FAT | PROTEIN | CARBS |
|------|------|---------|---------|-------|
| 322 | 15.8g | 3.5g | 10.4g | 29.4g |

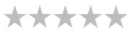

★★★★★

*Swapped the berries with bananas and used cow's milk.*
*Good-quality maple syrup elevates this from breakfast*
*to a comfort food.* **HA**

● EASY ○ FAMILY-FRIENDLY ○ GLUTEN FREE ● LOW CAL ○ QUICK ● VEGAN

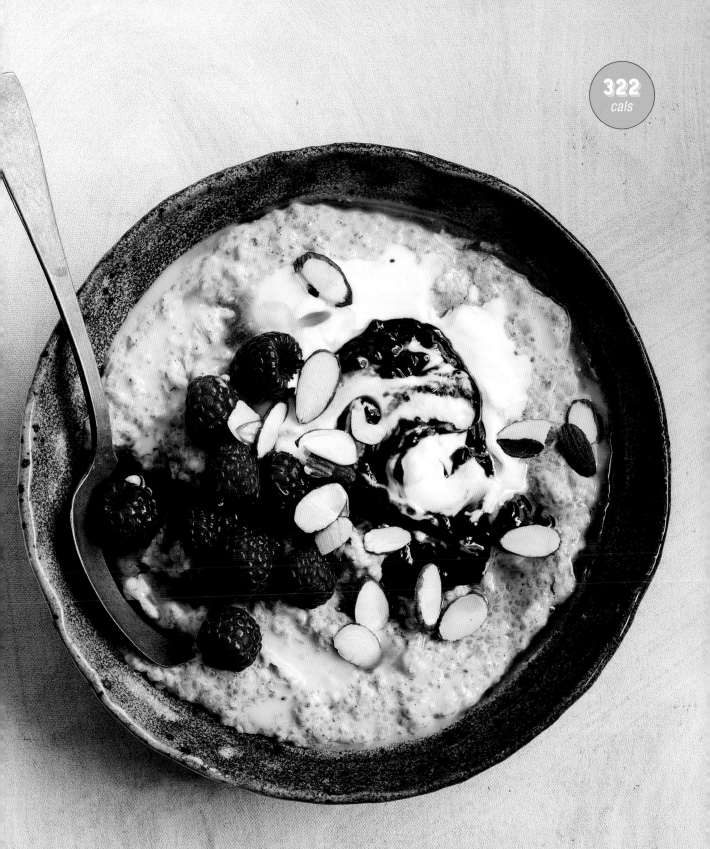

322
cals

35

# PUNCHY PROTEIN BREAKFAST
# BOWL

Ready in just 10 minutes, you'll love this combo of flavours
with the added protein of quinoa and a runny soft-boiled egg.

**SERVES** 1  **PREP** 5 mins  **COOK** 5 mins

1 egg
75g (½ cup) cooked quinoa, warmed
50g baby spinach
¼ avocado, sliced
1 tsp fresh lemon juice
1 tsp extra virgin olive oil
2 tsp chopped roasted unsalted
  almonds

**1** Place the egg in a small saucepan of cold water. Bring to the boil over high heat. Reduce heat to medium and gently boil, uncovered, stirring occasionally, for 4-5 minutes for a soft-boiled egg. Drain, then cool under cold running water. Peel and halve crossways.

**2** Arrange the quinoa, spinach, egg and avocado in a serving bowl. Drizzle over lemon juice and olive oil. Sprinkle with almond, to serve.

**COOK'S NOTE**

Cook a big batch of quinoa and keep in the fridge for up to 1 week. Simply reheat in the microwave before using.

## NUTRITION (PER SERVE)

| CALS | FAT | SAT FAT | PROTEIN | CARBS |
|------|-----|---------|---------|-------|
| 341.7 | 27.6g | 4.3g | 23.1g | 60.5g |

★★★★★

*Thank you for this recipe. It is wonderful to sit down on a weekend morning and slowly enjoy spoonfuls of quinoa and avo dripping in runny egg. Love it.* **SHAWNTHEPRAWN**

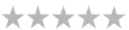

● EASY   ○ FAMILY-FRIENDLY   ● GLUTEN FREE   ● LOW CAL   ● QUICK   ○ VEGAN

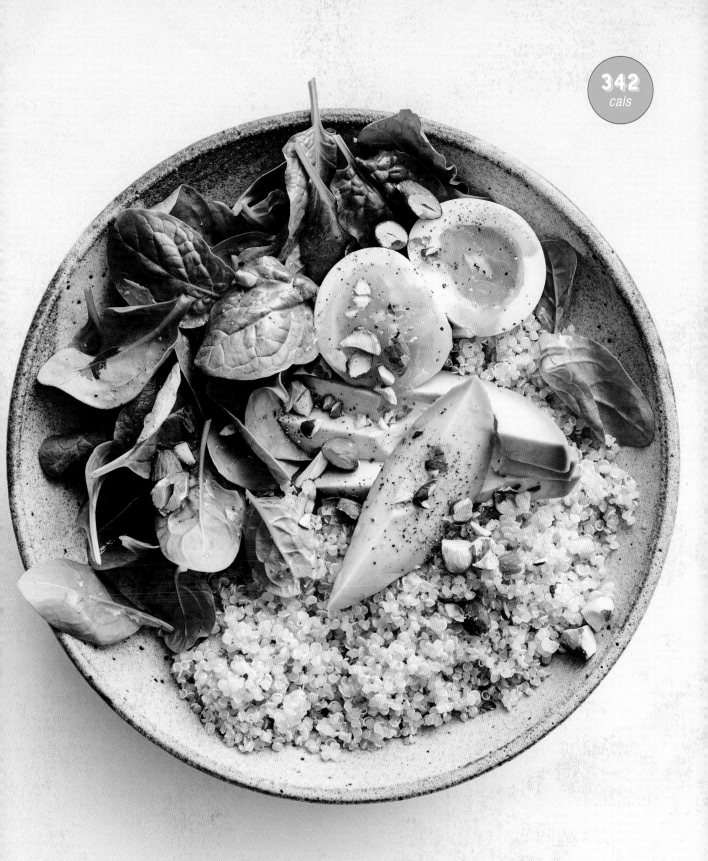

# CRISPIEST SWEETCORN FRITTERS

How did we make these easy corn fritters super crispy? We cooked them with a little cheese! Serve them with salsa for an extra boost of nutrients.

**MAKES** 16  **PREP** 10 mins  **COOK** 20 mins

420g can corn kernels,
  drained, rinsed
1 tbs chopped fresh chives,
  plus extra, to serve
200g haloumi, grated
80g (1 cup) grated cheddar
150g (1 cup) plain flour
1 tsp all purpose seasoning
180ml (¾ cup) milk
Rice bran oil, to shallow fry
Chopped tomato and firm
  ripe avocado, to serve

1 Combine the corn, chives, half the haloumi, half the cheddar, flour and seasoning in a bowl. Add the milk and stir to combine. Combine the remaining haloumi and cheddar in a separate bowl.

2 Fill a large deep frying pan with enough oil to come 1cm up side of pan. Place over medium-high heat. Working in batches, scoop ¼ cup batter into the pan for each fritter and flatten slightly. Cook for 2 minutes or until the underside is golden.

3 Spoon a little cheese mixture on top of each fritter and push lightly with the back of the spoon to secure. Turn over and cook for 2 minutes or until cooked through and golden. Transfer to a plate and cover to keep warm.

4 Combine the tomato and avocado in a serving bowl. Stack the fritters on a serving plate. Sprinkle fritters and tomato salsa with sea salt and chives. Serve.

**COOK'S NOTE**

Serve fritters for brunch with an egg on top, if you like. Keep uneaten fritters in an airtight container in the fridge for up to 3 days. Reheat, before serving.

## NUTRITION (PER 2 FRITTERS)

| CALS | FAT | SAT FAT | PROTEIN | CARBS |
|------|-----|---------|---------|-------|
| 306 | 18.5g | 7.5g | 11.9g | 21.25g |

● EASY  ● FAMILY-FRIENDLY  ○ GLUTEN FREE  ● LOW CAL  ● QUICK  ○ VEGAN

306
cals

★ ★ ★ ★ ★

*Very simple recipe. Will definitely try again. Family favourite!* **CLEMLEV222**

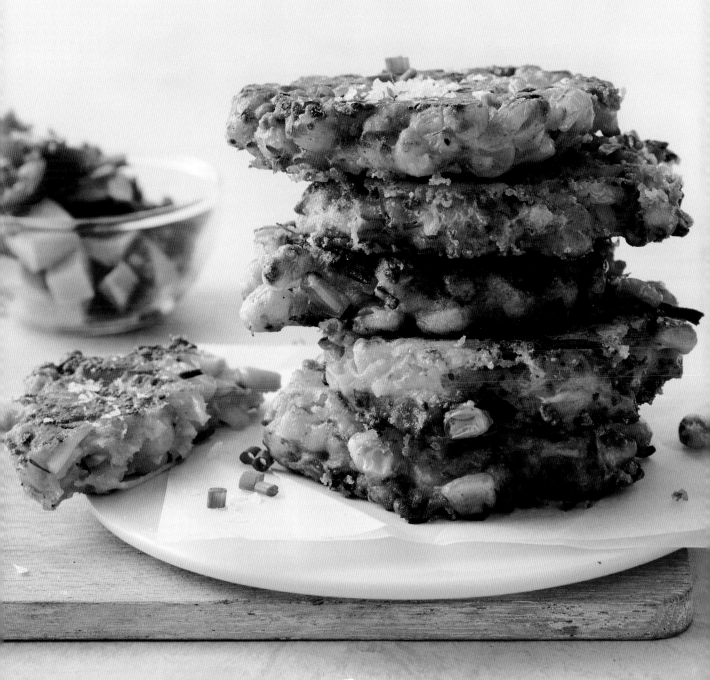

# HEALTHY BANANA WAFFLES

For a simple low-cal brekky, you can't go past our healthy banana and oat waffles topped with yoghurt and mixed berries.

**SERVES** 4 **PREP** 5 mins **COOK** 5 mins

150g rolled oats
1 large banana
2 tsp baking powder
1 tsp ground cinnamon
125ml (½ cup) unsweetened almond milk
2 eggs
130g (½ cup) natural yoghurt
130g (1 cup) frozen mixed berries, thawed
Honey, to drizzle (optional)

1 Place the oats in a food processor and process until finely ground (like flour). Add the banana, baking powder, cinnamon, almond milk and eggs. Process until mixture is smooth.

2 Preheat a waffle iron. Lightly spray with oil. Ladle one-quarter of oat mixture into each hole. Close the lid. Cook for 1-2 minutes or until waffles are golden. Repeat with the remaining mixture, if needed (depends on the size of your waffle iron), to make 4 waffles in total.

3 Serve waffles topped with yoghurt, berries and a drizzle of honey, if desired.

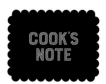

**COOK'S NOTE**

Swap the frozen berries for fresh individual or mixed berries, if you like.

## NUTRITION (PER SERVE)

| CALS | FAT | SAT FAT | PROTEIN | CARBS |
|------|------|---------|---------|-------|
| 285 | 10.6g | 3.5g | 11.7g | 30.9g |

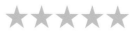

*Yum! I used half milk and half Greek yoghurt to make them a bit lighter, and they came out beautiful and fluffy. So good.* **ANNAJW**

● EASY ○ FAMILY-FRIENDLY ○ GLUTEN FREE ● LOW CAL ● QUICK ○ VEGAN

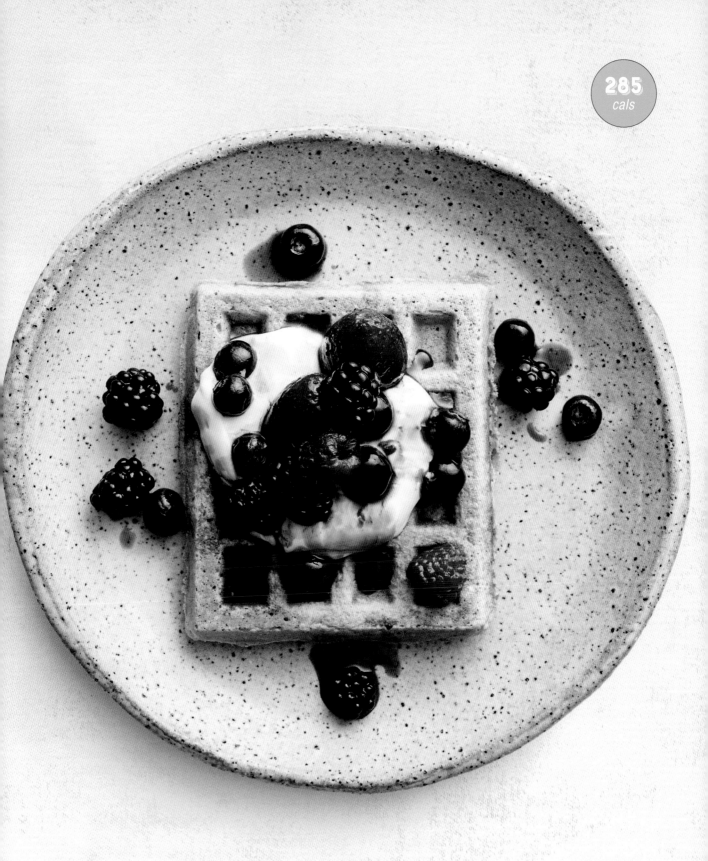

285
*cals*

# CHOC, FRUIT & OAT BREKKY BOWL

You'll be bowled over by this yummy combo. Be sure to prep it the night before so the oats soak up the chocolate and vanilla flavours.

**SERVES** 4 **PREP** 5 mins (+ overnight soaking) **COOK** 5 mins

125g (1⅓ cups) rolled oats
55g (⅓ cup) white chia seeds
2 tbs raw cacao powder or
   dark cocoa powder
750ml (3 cups) milk
1 tbs maple syrup
1 tsp vanilla extract
25g (⅓ cup) dried coconut chips
1 tbs pistachio kernels
260g (1 cup) no-added-sugar
   vanilla yoghurt
2 figs, cut into wedges
12 strawberries, hulled, halved
12 raspberries, halved
Beetroot powder, to dust
   (optional, see note)
Fresh mint sprigs and edible
   flowers (optional), to serve

**1** Place the oats, chia seeds and cacao or cocoa powder in a bowl. Add the milk, maple syrup and vanilla, and stir to combine. Cover with plastic wrap and place in the fridge to soak overnight.

**2** Place coconut chips in a frying pan over medium heat. Cook, stirring, for 1 minute or until toasted. Transfer to a plate. Add the pistachios to the pan. Cook, stirring, for 2 minutes or until toasted. Transfer to a plate. Set aside to cool, before coarsely chopping.

**3** Divide the oat mixture between serving bowls. Top with yoghurt, fig, strawberry, raspberry, toasted coconut and pistachio. Add mint and the edible flowers, if using. Dust yoghurt with beetroot powder, if you like, then serve.

**COOK'S NOTE**

Natural beetroot powder is rich in nitrates and is known to improve blood circulation. Pick it up at health food stores and chemists.

## NUTRITION (PER SERVE)

| CALS | FAT | SAT FAT | PROTEIN | CARBS |
|------|-----|---------|---------|-------|
| 398 | 15g | 4.9g | 17.5g | 20g |

★★★★★

*Easy to prep the night before. I didn't bother toasting the coconut and oats, so putting it all together in the morning was quick.* **BLYMER**

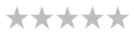

○ EASY   ○ FAMILY-FRIENDLY   ○ GLUTEN FREE   ● LOW CAL   ○ QUICK   ○ VEGAN

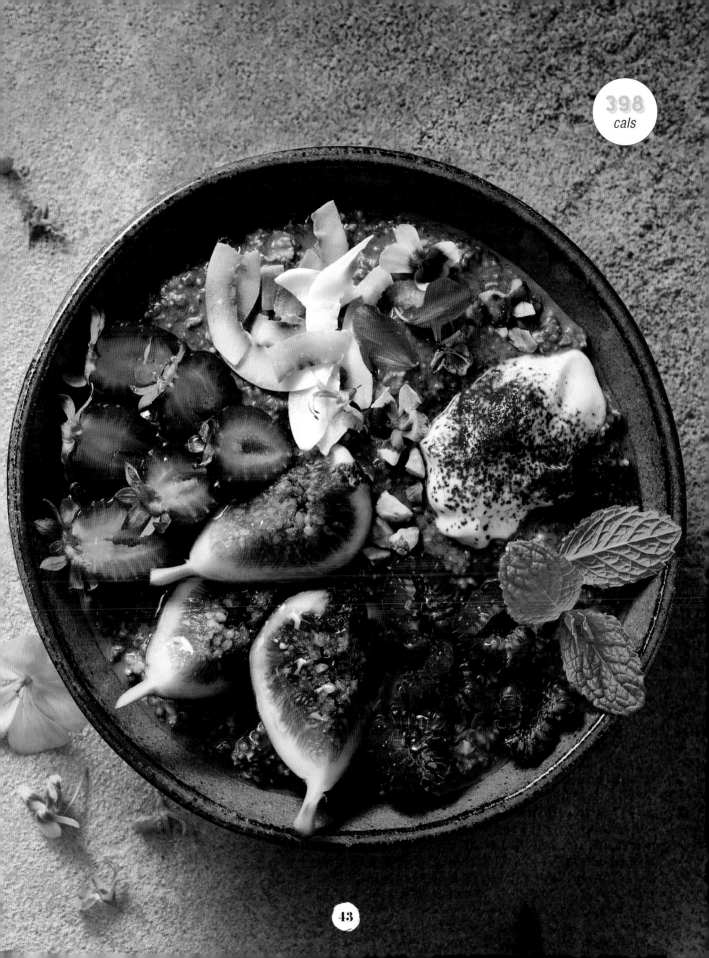

# ONE-PAN SWEET POTATO & EGG HASH

This beautifully bright breakfast is a hearty healthy twist on your regular potato hash – plus, it's quick and easy. You can make it with leftover veg, too.

**SERVES** 4  **PREP** 10 mins  **COOK** 25 mins

1 tbs extra virgin olive oil
1 red onion, finely chopped
600g sweet potato, peeled, cut into 1.5cm pieces
1 red capsicum, deseeded, finely chopped
2 garlic cloves, crushed
2 zucchini, cut into 1cm pieces
4 eggs
¼ cup fresh basil leaves
Pinch of dried chilli flakes (optional)

1 Heat the oil in a large non-stick frying pan over medium-high heat. Add the onion and cook, stirring often, for 3-4 minutes or until golden.

2 Add the sweet potato, capsicum and garlic. Cook, stirring occasionally, for 10 minutes or until golden. Add the zucchini. Cover and cook for 5 minutes or until all vegetables are tender.

3 Make 4 indents in the vegetable mixture and crack an egg into each indent. Cover and cook for 4-5 minutes, or until the eggs are cooked to your liking. Serve sprinkled with basil and the chilli flakes, if using.

**COOK'S NOTE**

Use any leftover cooked vegies you have on hand, such as pumpkin or potato. You could also add some crumbled feta, if you like.

## NUTRITION (PER SERVE)

| CALS | FAT | SAT FAT | PROTEIN | CARBS |
|------|-----|---------|---------|-------|
| 248 | 9.6g | 1.9g | 11.8g | 25.4g |

★★★★★ *This is a delicious vegie-filled breakfast that I have made numerous times! I halve the recipe as there are only two of us and add paprika to the vegies while they are cooking for a bit of extra flavour. Serve with chilli jam and basil, yum!* **GRILLEDSANDWICH**

● EASY  ○ FAMILY-FRIENDLY  ● GLUTEN FREE  ● LOW CAL  ○ QUICK  ○ VEGAN

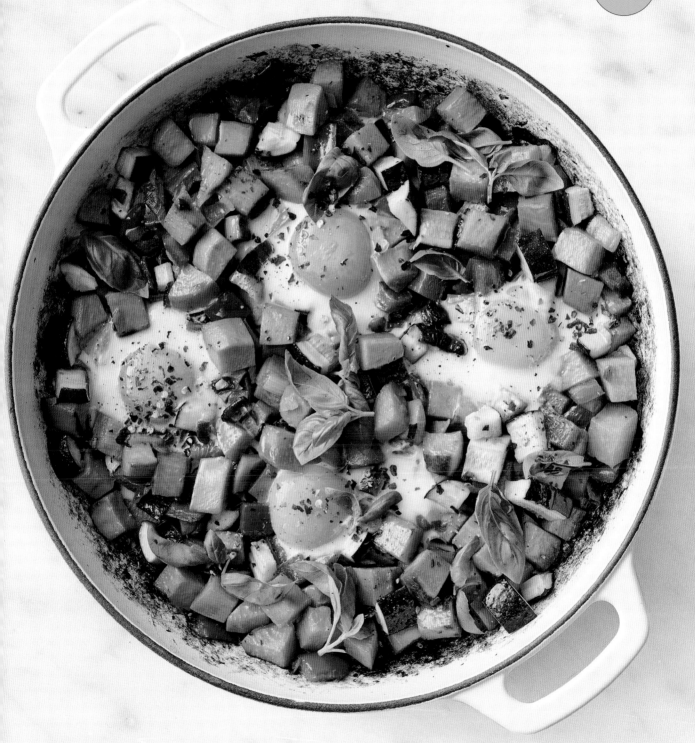

# PUMPKIN & BASIL
# RISOTTO

Get your fill with this sweet and creamy risotto cleverly served in pumpkin-shell bowls. It's a recipe the whole family will savour.

**SERVES** 6 **PREP** 15 mins **COOK** 1 hour 10 mins

1.8kg butternut pumpkin, halved, deseeded
2 tbs extra virgin olive oil
750ml (3 cups) gluten-free chicken stock
1 brown onion, finely chopped
2 garlic cloves, thinly sliced
220g (1 cup) arborio rice
160ml (⅔ cup) white wine
70g (1 cup) finely grated parmesan
1 cup fresh basil leaves, chopped
100g (1 cup) coarsely grated mozzarella
Salad leaves, to serve (optional)

1 Preheat oven to 200°C/180°C fan forced. Place pumpkin, cut-side up, on a baking tray. Use a sharp knife to deeply score flesh in a crisscross pattern, leaving a 2-3cm border. Drizzle with 1 tbs oil. Bake for 50 minutes or until tender.

2 Meanwhile, place the stock in a saucepan over high heat. Bring just to the boil. Reduce heat to low. Hold at a gentle simmer.

3 Heat the remaining oil in a saucepan over medium heat. Cook the onion and garlic, stirring, for 5 minutes or until softened. Stir in the rice for 1 minute or until slightly translucent. Add wine. Cook, stirring, until liquid is absorbed. Add enough stock to just cover the rice. Stir until absorbed. Continue adding stock to just cover the rice, stirring constantly and allowing liquid to absorb before adding more, for 18 minutes or until rice is tender yet firm to the bite.

4 Use a large metal spoon to scoop out the cooked pumpkin flesh, leaving the border. Coarsely chop and stir into the risotto with the parmesan and basil. Season.

5 Fill pumpkin halves with risotto. Sprinkle with the mozzarella. Bake for 20 minutes or until cheese is golden and melted. Serve.

**COOK'S NOTE**

To add some greens, stir baby spinach leaves into the risotto at the end of step 4.

## NUTRITION (PER SERVE)

| CALS | FAT | SAT FAT | PROTEIN | CARBS |
|------|------|---------|---------|-------|
| 397 | 13.7g | 4.8g | 13.4g | 47g |

● EASY  ● FAMILY-FRIENDLY  ● GLUTEN FREE  ● LOW CAL  ○ QUICK  ○ VEGAN

397 cals

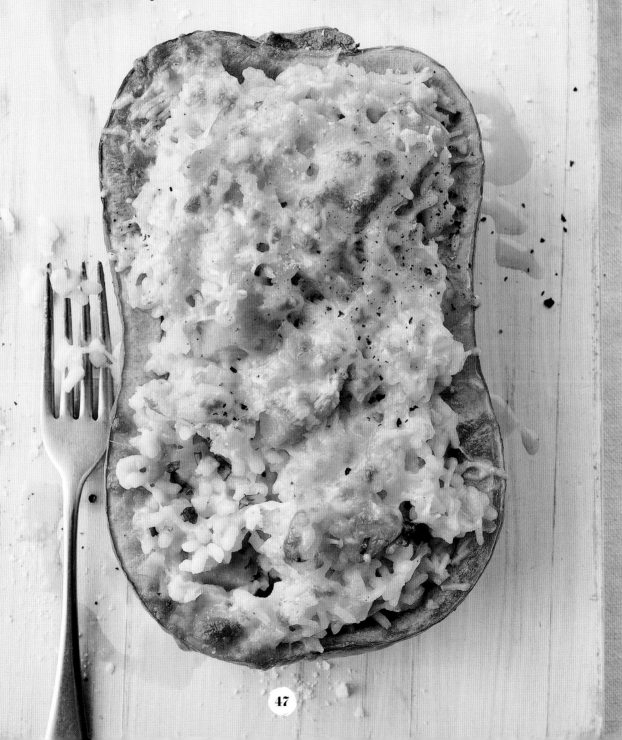

# HEALTHY LEEK & BROCCOLI SOUP

Fight coughs and colds with this healthy soup. It contains a whole leek, which is a natural prebiotic, and nutrient-stacked broccoli.

**SERVES** 4  **PREP** 15 mins  **COOK** 25 mins

1 tbs extra virgin olive oil, plus extra, to serve
1 large leek, white part only, thinly sliced
2 large celery sticks, pale leaves reserved, finely chopped
2 garlic cloves, crushed
2 tsp finely grated lemon rind
2 (about 300g) potatoes, peeled, chopped
500ml (2 cups) salt-reduced, gluten-free vegetable stock
500ml (2 cups) water
1 large zucchini, chopped
450g broccoli, cut into florets
75g baby spinach
50g creamy feta, crumbled
1 tbs pepitas, toasted

1 Heat the oil in a large saucepan over medium heat. Add the leek and celery. Cook, stirring, for 6-7 minutes or until softened. Add the garlic and lemon rind. Cook, stirring, for 1 minute or until aromatic. Add the potato, stock and water. Bring to the boil. Reduce the heat to low, partially cover, and simmer for 5 minutes. Add the zucchini and broccoli. Simmer, partially covered, for 6-7 minutes or until the broccoli is tender. Stir in the spinach until just wilted.

2 Use a stick blender to blend soup in the pan until smooth. Season. Top with feta, pepitas, reserved celery leaves and a drizzle of extra oil. Season with black pepper. Serve.

**COOK'S NOTE**

Always use the broccoli stems as well as the florets. They are delicious and a valuable source of fibre.

## NUTRITION (PER SERVE)

| CALS | FAT | SAT FAT | PROTEIN | CARBS |
|------|-----|---------|---------|-------|
| 208 | 9.5g | 3g | 12.5g | 13g |

● EASY  ● FAMILY-FRIENDLY  ● GLUTEN FREE  ● LOW CAL  ○ QUICK  ○ VEGAN

208
cals

★ ★ ★ ★ ★
*We loved this. Every mouthful has something new, different, whether it was melted feta or the roasted pepitas, or a hit of garlic. So easy and tasty. Definitely will make this again.* **CORRMAGS**

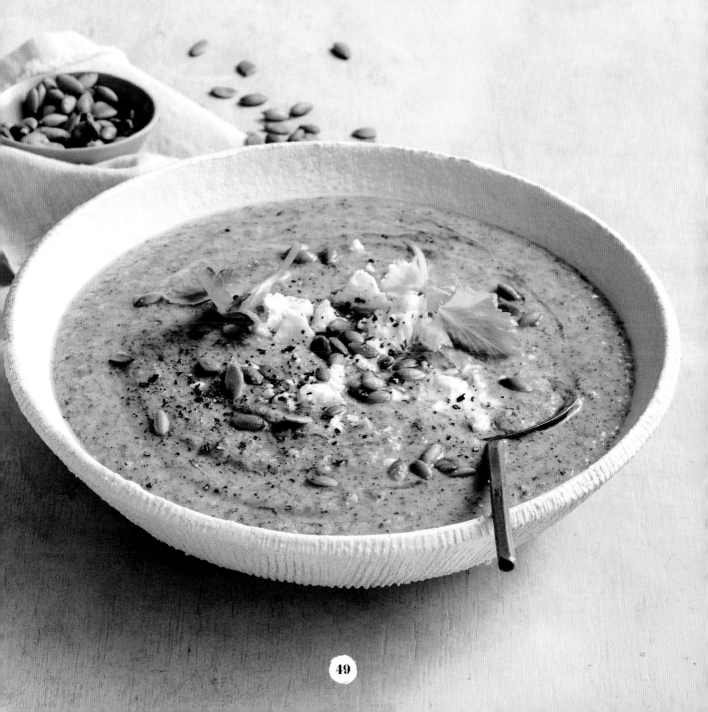

# ZUCCHINI & HALOUMI QUICHE

With delightfully flaky filo pastry, two types of cheese and vitamin-rich zucchini, this easy quiche recipe makes for a substantial lunch.

**SERVES** 8  **PREP** 20 mins  **COOK** 1 hour 20 mins

1 tbs olive oil
6 green shallots, chopped
2 large garlic cloves, crushed
5 (about 550g) medium zucchini
120g haloumi, grated, plus extra 60g, sliced
40g (½ cup) grated cheddar
8 eggs
180ml (¾ cup) thickened cream
12 sheets fresh filo pastry
100g butter, melted
2 tbs pomegranate arils

1. Preheat oven to 180°C/160°C fan forced. Lightly grease a 22cm springform pan. Combine the oil, shallot and garlic in a small frying pan over medium-low heat. Cook, stirring, for 3-4 minutes or until softened. Transfer to a large bowl.

2. Coarsely grate 3 zucchini. Use hands to squeeze out excess liquid. Add to the bowl. Stir in grated haloumi and cheddar. Whisk eggs and cream in a jug.

3. Place filo on a clean work surface. Cover with a dry tea towel then a damp tea towel (to prevent drying). Brush 1 filo sheet with a little melted butter. Top with another sheet at right angles. Brush with butter. Place another sheet diagonally on top. Brush with butter. Top with another at right angles to the last. Brush with butter. Repeat, layering in the same pattern with the remaining filo sheets and butter.

4. Carefully transfer filo stack to the prepared pan, pushing gently to shape to the pan. Stir egg mixture into the zucchini mixture and season with pepper. Pour into filo case. Trim overhanging filo. Fold pastry edge inwards to form a rim level with the top of the pan (the filling won't come right to the top at this stage).

5. Place pan on a baking tray. Bake for 1 hour 10 minutes or until filling is set and pastry is golden. Cool to room temperature. Use a vegetable peeler to slice remaining zucchini lengthways into ribbons. Spray with oil. Heat a chargrill pan over medium-high heat. Add zucchini and sliced haloumi. Cook, turning, for 1-2 minutes or until lightly charred.

6. Top quiche with zucchini and haloumi. Sprinkle with pomegranate. Cut the quiche into wedges, to serve.

## NUTRITION (PER SERVE)

| CALS | FAT | SAT FAT | PROTEIN | CARBS |
|------|-----|---------|---------|-------|
| 307 | 24g | 13.6g | 5.8g | 38.9g |

○ EASY  ● **FAMILY-FRIENDLY**  ○ GLUTEN FREE  ● **LOW CAL**  ○ QUICK  ○ VEGAN

307 cals

★ ★ ★ ★ ★

*I made this for a picnic brunch with the girls. So much flavour, especially if you add the little pops of pomegranate.* **CURLYSHIRLEY**

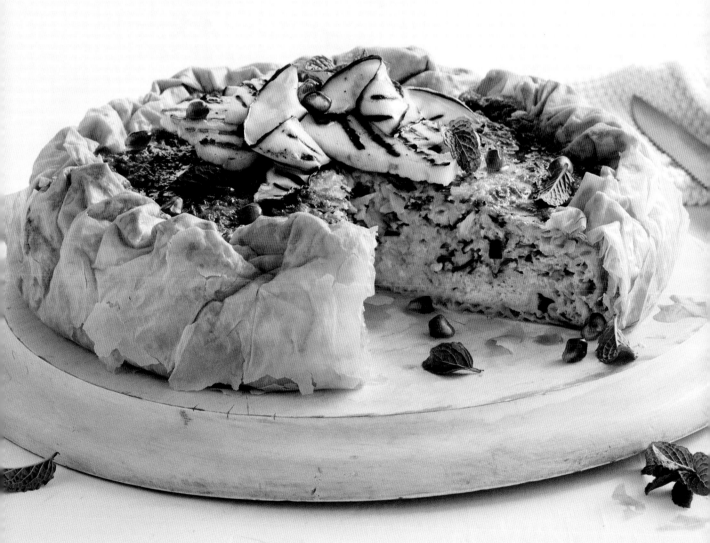

# PUMPKIN CURRY WITH TOFU

This low-cal curry is packed with tofu, which is high in protein and phytonutrients, pumpkin and beans to prove you can eat hearty yet healthy.

**SERVES** 4  **PREP** 20 mins  **COOK** 30 mins

1 large onion, chopped
2 garlic cloves, crushed
1 tbs finely grated fresh ginger
2 long fresh red chillies, deseeded, chopped
2 tsp curry powder
2 tsp macadamia oil
350g firm tofu, cut into cubes
12 fresh curry leaves, plus extra, fried, to serve
300ml reduced-fat coconut milk
300ml salt-reduced, gluten-free vegetable stock
500g pumpkin, peeled, deseeded, cut into 3cm pieces
200g green beans, trimmed, halved
75g baby spinach
300g (2 cups) cooked quinoa
Lime halves, to serve

**1** Place the onion, garlic, ginger, chilli and curry powder in a small food processor. Process until a thick paste forms.

**2** Heat half the oil in a large wok or non-stick frying pan over high heat. Cook the tofu, in 2 batches, stirring, for 2-3 minutes or until golden. Transfer to a plate and set aside.

**3** Reduce heat to medium. Add the curry paste to the wok. Cook, stirring, for 3-4 minutes or until aromatic. Add the curry leaves. Cook, stirring, for 1 minute.

**4** Pour in the coconut milk and stock. Bring to the boil. Reduce the heat to low and simmer, covered, for 5 minutes. Add the pumpkin and tofu. Simmer, covered, for 6-7 minutes or until the pumpkin is almost tender. Add the beans. Simmer, covered, for 2-3 minutes or until tender. Stir in the spinach until just wilted.

**5** Divide quinoa among serving plates. Top with the curry and extra curry leaves. Serve with lime halves to squeeze.

### COOK'S NOTE

Use any of your favourite vegies in this dish – cauliflower, eggplant, sweet potato or mushrooms would all be delicious.

## NUTRITION (PER SERVE)

| CALS | FAT | SAT FAT | PROTEIN | CARBS |
|------|-----|---------|---------|-------|
| 391 | 17g | 6g | 20g | 32.5g |

★★★★★ *Love it, super easy. I used 400ml coconut milk and it was fine. I didn't blitz the ingredients, just threw them in grated.* **USER_17783**

○ EASY   ○ FAMILY-FRIENDLY   ● **GLUTEN FREE**   ● **LOW CAL**   ○ QUICK   ● **VEGAN**

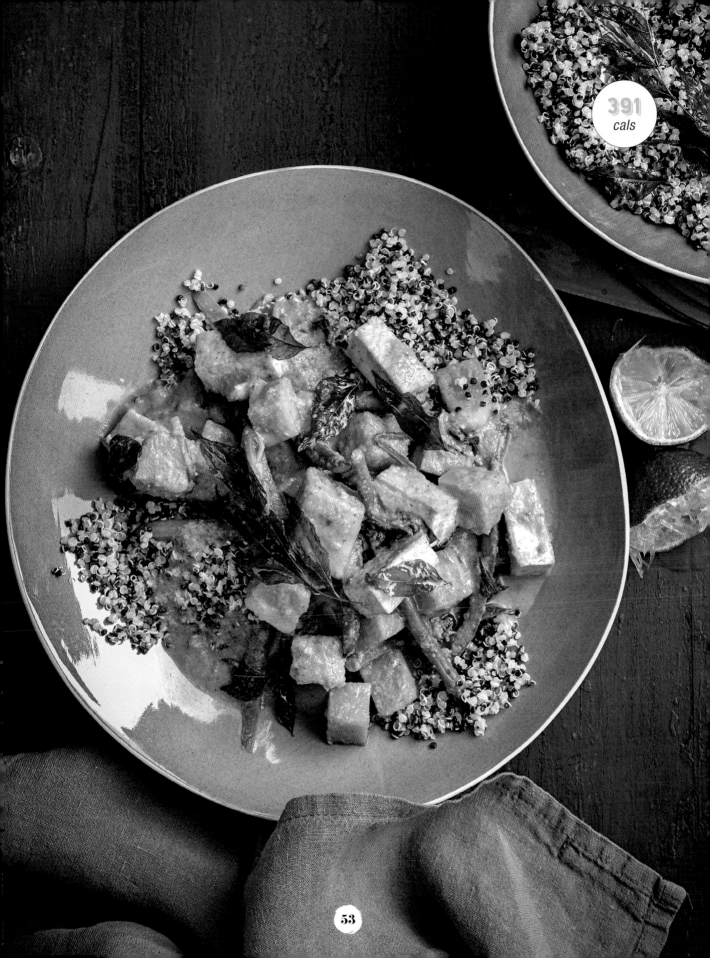

391
*cals*

# 'VEGTASTIC'

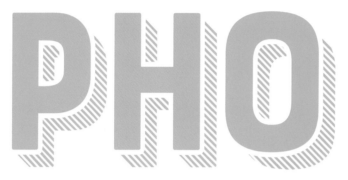

# PHO

Everyone's favourite Vietnamese rice noodle soup – pho – is now vegetarian. Our slow cooked version is every bit as soul-soothing as the meaty one.

**SERVES** 4  **PREP** 10 mins  **COOK** 4 hours 20 mins

250g rice vermicelli noodles
Light soy sauce, to taste
1 bunch baby pak choy, quartered
   lengthways
300g firm tofu, cut into 1.5cm pieces
Bean sprouts, fresh Vietnamese mint
   sprigs, sliced fresh red chilli,
   hot chilli sauce and lime wedges,
   to serve

**VEGETABLE BROTH**
2 cinnamon sticks
2 whole star anise
5 cloves
1½ tsp coriander seeds
1 tsp black peppercorns
1 large brown onion, quartered
5cm-piece ginger, peeled, halved
   horizontally
20g (¾ cup) sliced, dried shiitake
   mushrooms
3L (12 cups) gluten-free
   vegetable stock

1 To make the broth, place the cinnamon, star anise, cloves, coriander seeds and peppercorns in a frying pan over medium heat. Cook, shaking the pan occasionally, for 2-3 minutes or until aromatic. Set aside to cool slightly. Transfer spices to a piece of muslin and tie with kitchen string to make a bouquet garni. Set aside. Add onion and ginger to the frying pan. Cook, stirring, for 3-5 minutes or until lightly charred.

2 Place the onion mixture, bouquet garni and mushroom in a 6L slow cooker. Add the stock. Cover and cook on High for 4 hours.

3 Five minutes before the broth is ready, place the noodles in a large heatproof bowl and cover with boiling water. Set aside for 5 minutes to soften. Drain well. Remove spice pouch from broth. Stir in soy sauce, to taste.

4 Add the pak choy and tofu to the slow cooker. Cover. Cook on High for 5-10 minutes or until the pak choy is tender. Divide the noodles and soup among serving bowls. Top with bean sprouts, mint and sliced chilli. Serve with chilli sauce and lime wedges.

## NUTRITION (PER SERVE)

| CALS | FAT | SAT FAT | PROTEIN | CARBS |
|------|-----|---------|---------|-------|
| 365  | 8g  | 2g      | 17g     | 52g   |

○ EASY   ○ FAMILY-FRIENDLY   ● GLUTEN FREE   ● LOW CAL   ○ QUICK   ● VEGAN

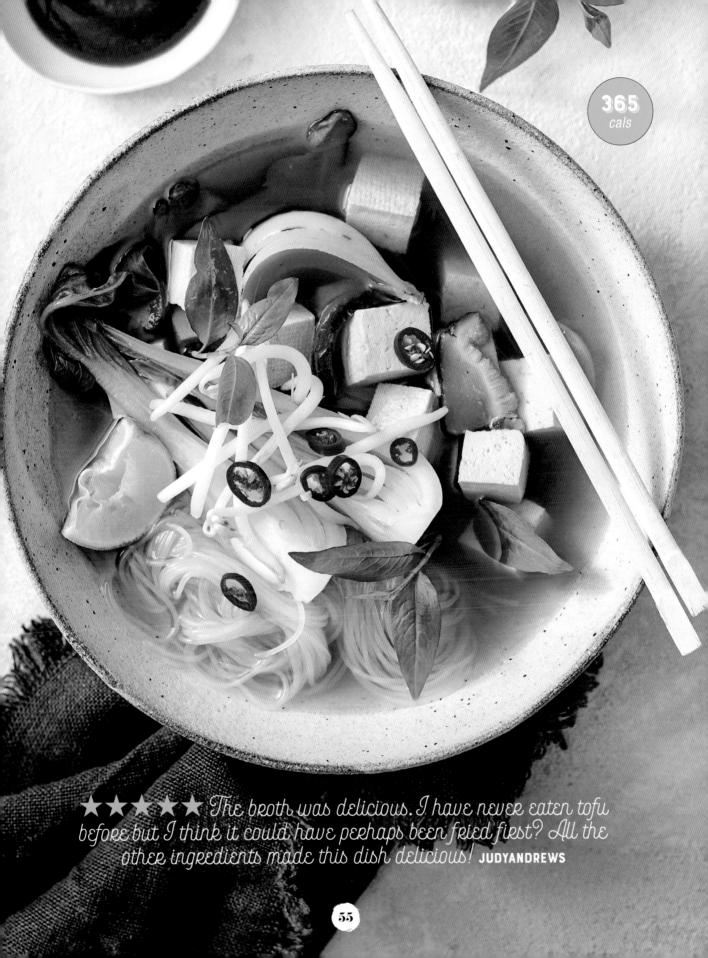

★★★★★ The broth was delicious. I have never eaten tofu before but I think it could have perhaps been fried first? All the other ingredients made this dish delicious! JUDYANDREWS

365 cals

# TOFU, CORN & MUNG BEAN SALSA

Dress up grilled tofu with this spicy, zesty Mexican-inspired vegan dish. The crunchy mung beans and corn, and creamy avo, are simply 'salsational'!

**SERVES** 4 **PREP** 20 mins (+ 1 hour marinating) **COOK** 15 mins

2 tsp chipotle sauce
1 tbs no-added-salt tomato paste
1 tbs salt-reduced, gluten-free tamari
350g firm tofu, cut into 8 slices
3 large corncobs, husks removed
200g pkt fresh mung bean sprouts, rinsed, drained (see note)
1 cup fresh coriander leaves
½ firm ripe avocado, chopped
1 long fresh green chilli, deseeded, sliced
1 tbs lime juice
2 tsp extra virgin olive oil
4 small gluten-free corn tortillas, grilled, to serve
Lime wedges, to serve

1 Combine the chipotle sauce, tomato paste and tamari in a shallow glass or ceramic dish. Add the tofu and turn to coat. Cover. Place in the fridge for 1 hour to marinate.

2 Preheat a chargrill or barbecue grill on medium-high. Spray the corn with oil and add to the grill. Cook, turning, for 8-10 minutes, or until lightly charred and tender. Transfer to a plate. Add tofu to the grill. Cook for 2 minutes each side or until lightly charred and golden. Transfer to the plate.

3 Use a sharp knife to remove kernels from the cob. Combine the kernels, mung beans, coriander, avocado and chilli in a bowl. Whisk the lime juice and olive oil in a jug and add to the corn mixture. Toss to combine.

4 Divide corn salsa and tofu among serving plates. Serve with the tortillas and lime wedges.

**COOK'S NOTE**

Mung beans are small legumes that are rich in protein, folate and vitamins. They add delicious crunch to this recipe.

## NUTRITION (PER SERVE)

| CALS | FAT | SAT FAT | PROTEIN | CARBS |
|------|-----|---------|---------|-------|
| 368 | 18g | 3g | 19g | 25g |

○ EASY  ○ FAMILY-FRIENDLY  ● GLUTEN FREE  ● LOW CAL  ○ QUICK  ● VEGAN

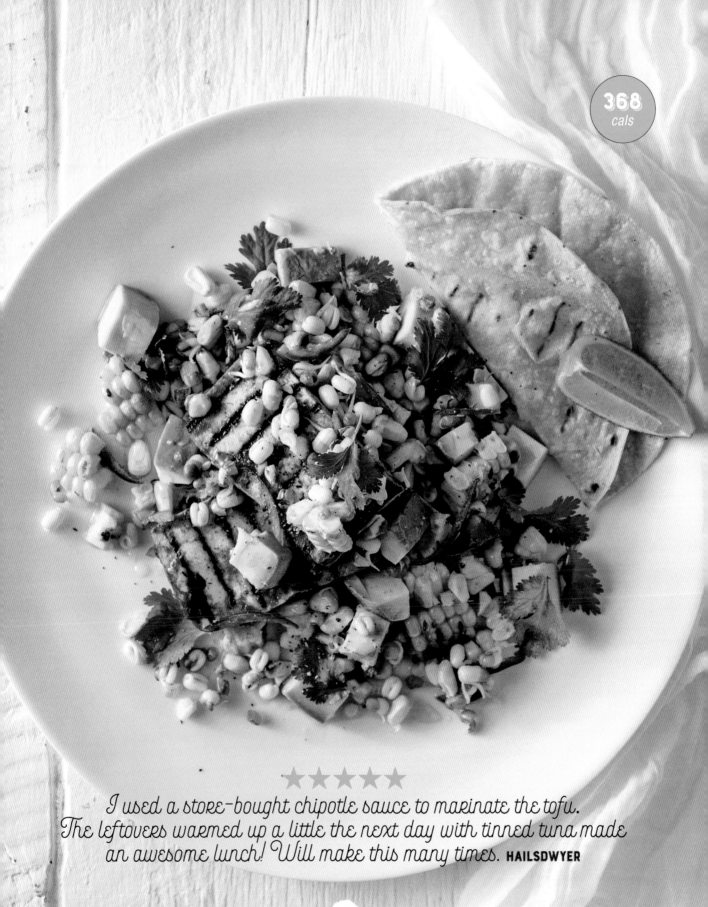

368 cals

★★★★★

*I used a store-bought chipotle sauce to marinate the tofu. The leftovers warmed up a little the next day with tinned tuna made an awesome lunch! Will make this many times.* **HAILSDWYER**

# LENTIL, BRUSSELS & MUSHIE
# MEDLEY

It's roasted perfection on a plate! Such a good mix of fibre, protein, vitamins and antioxidants doesn't come much more delicious than this.

**SERVES** 4  **PREP** 15 mins  **COOK** 35 mins

250g brussels sprouts, trimmed, halved

2 eschalots, cut into wedges

2½ tbs extra virgin olive oil

4 large portobello mushrooms

25g butter, finely chopped

1 tsp fresh thyme leaves

105g (½ cup) dried green puy lentils, washed

70g (½ cup) pecans, halved

1 small radicchio, leaves torn (see note)

1 garlic clove, thinly sliced

2 tbs cider vinegar

2 tbs chopped fresh continental parsley leaves, plus extra, to serve

1 Preheat oven to 220°C/200°C fan forced. Line 2 large baking trays with baking paper.

2 Place brussels sprouts and eschalot on 1 prepared tray. Drizzle with 1 tbs oil. Season. Place the mushrooms on the second prepared tray, stem-side up. Drizzle with 1 tbs remaining oil and top with butter pieces. Sprinkle with the thyme. Season.

3 Roast vegetables for 25 minutes or until the brussels sprouts are golden and crisp, and the mushrooms are tender with a buttery sauce formed inside.

4 Meanwhile, cook the lentils following packet directions. Drain. Set aside. Heat remaining oil in a large frying pan. Add the pecans and cook, stirring, for 2 minutes or until toasted. Add the radicchio and garlic. Cook, tossing occasionally, for 3-4 minutes or until radicchio just starts to wilt. Add lentils, brussels sprouts and eschalot. Drizzle with vinegar. Season. Toss to combine. Stir in parsley.

5 Spoon lentil mixture onto serving plates. Top each with a mushroom, keeping butter sauce inside. Serve sprinkled with extra parsley.

## COOK'S NOTE

You can use red cabbage or witlof instead of the radicchio, if you like.

## NUTRITION (PER SERVE)

| CALS | FAT | SAT FAT | PROTEIN | CARBS |
|---|---|---|---|---|
| 373 | 27.4g | 5.7g | 11.8g | 10.7g |

○ EASY  ○ FAMILY-FRIENDLY  ● GLUTEN FREE  ● LOW CAL  ○ QUICK  ○ VEGAN

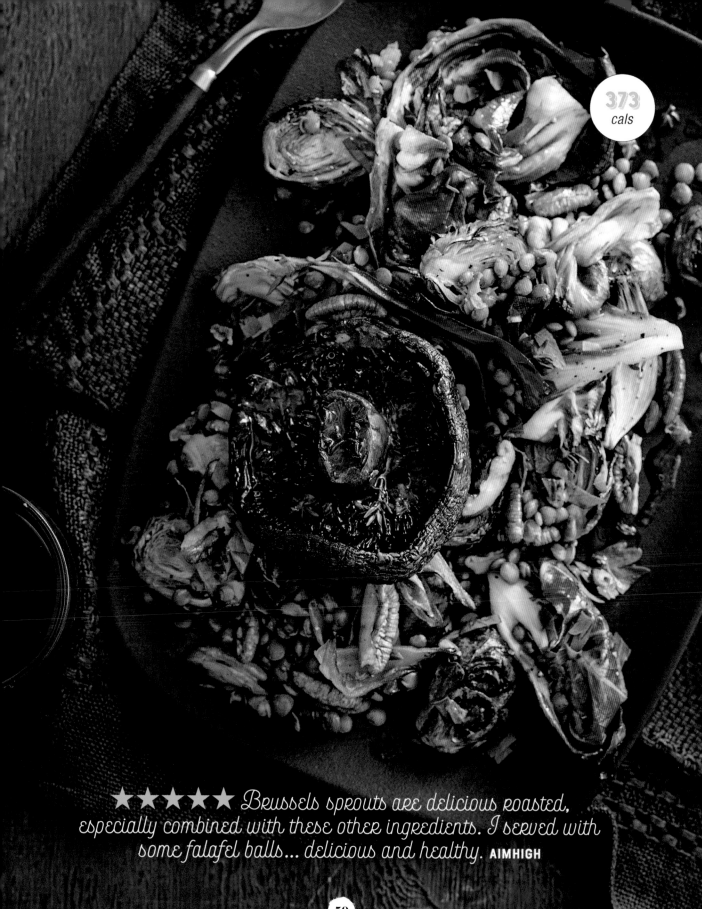

373 cals

★★★★★ Brussels sprouts are delicious roasted, especially combined with these other ingredients. I served with some falafel balls... delicious and healthy. **AIMHIGH**

# VEGETARIAN RAMEN
# BOWL

This easy ramen dinner bowl is jammed full with noodles, pumpkin and mushrooms. With a rich vegetable broth, it will warm you, too.

**SERVES** 4 **PREP** 15 mins **COOK** 20 mins

75g (¼ cup) white miso paste
80ml (¼ cup) light soy sauce
2 tsp honey
1 tsp vegetable oil
500g kent pumpkin, seeds removed, skin on, thinly sliced
4 eggs
1.5L (6 cups) vegetable stock
8 dried shiitake mushrooms
2 tsp finely grated fresh ginger
1 bunch baby bok choy, halved or quartered lengthways
2 small carrots, thinly sliced
450g shelf-fresh ramen noodles
2 green shallots, thinly sliced
2 tsp sesame seeds, toasted
Dried chilli flakes and thinly shredded nori, to serve (optional)

**1** Preheat oven to 200°C/180°C fan forced. Line a baking tray with baking paper. Use a fork to whisk 1 tbs miso paste, 1 tbs soy sauce, honey and oil in a jug.

**2** Arrange pumpkin slices on the prepared tray and brush with half the miso mixture. Turn over and brush the other side with remaining miso mixture. Roast for 15-20 minutes or until pumpkin is tender. Transfer to a plate.

**3** Meanwhile, place eggs in a saucepan and cover with water. Bring to the boil over high heat. As soon as the water boils, cook for 2 minutes. Drain and cool under cold running water. Peel and halve lengthways. Add to plate with pumpkin.

**4** Combine the stock, mushrooms, ginger and remaining soy sauce in a large saucepan. Cover and bring to a simmer over medium heat. Add the carrot and simmer for 2 minutes or until tender-crisp. Remove from heat and stir in the remaining miso paste until dissolved. Toss in the noodles and bok choy. Set aside for 2 minutes or until noodles are warmed through and bok choy is tender.

**5** Divide the soup among bowls. Top with pumpkin and egg, then sprinkle with shallot, sesame seeds, plus the chilli flakes and nori, if using.

## NUTRITION (PER SERVE)

| CALS | FAT | SAT FAT | PROTEIN | CARBS |
|------|-----|---------|---------|-------|
| 391 | 10.7g | 2.4g | 19.8g | 49.5g |

★★★★★

*Was absolutely amazing, sooo much flavour.* **MEGANWILSON95**

○ EASY   ○ FAMILY-FRIENDLY   ○ GLUTEN FREE   ● LOW CAL   ○ QUICK   ○ VEGAN

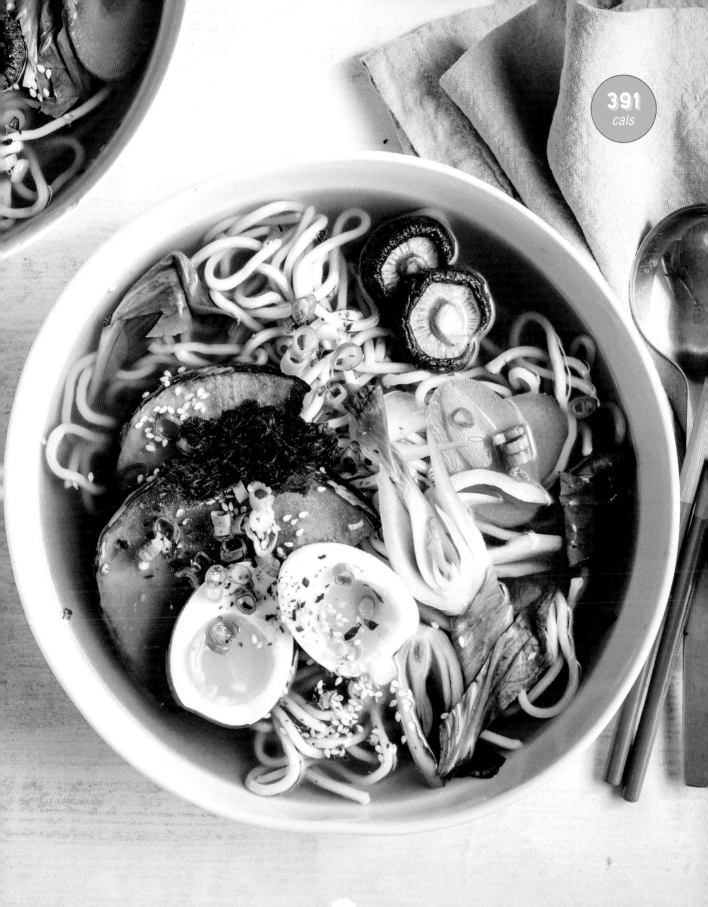

391
*cals*

# ONE-POT KETO ZUCCHINI
# ALFREDO

A real dinner winner, this creamy cheesy low-carb 'spaghetti' dish can be on the dining table in just 15 minutes. It's fast food the easy way.

**SERVES** 4 **PREP** 5 mins **COOK** 10 mins

1 tbs extra virgin olive oil
15g butter
2 x 250g pkt zucchini noodles
2 garlic cloves, finely chopped
100g cream cheese, chopped
1 tbs thickened cream
20g (¼ cup) finely grated parmesan,
   plus extra, to serve

**1** Heat the oil and butter in a frying pan over medium-high heat until butter is foamy. Add the zucchini noodles. Use tongs to toss occasionally for 1-2 minutes or until slightly wilted. Transfer to a plate.

**2** Add garlic to the pan. Cook, stirring, for 1 minute or until aromatic. Add the cream cheese, cream and 60ml (¼ cup) water. Reduce heat to low. Cook, stirring often, for 3 minutes or until smooth. Stir through the parmesan and season. Add the zucchini and toss to coat in the sauce. Serve immediately, sprinkled with extra parmesan.

### COOK'S NOTE

To up the vegie factor, toss steamed broccoli florets and green peas into the pan when you return the zucchini.

## NUTRITION (PER SERVE)

| CALS | FAT | SAT FAT | PROTEIN | CARBS |
|------|-----|---------|---------|-------|
| 232 | 21.4g | 11.3g | 7g | 2.5g |

● EASY  ○ FAMILY-FRIENDLY  ● GLUTEN FREE  ● LOW CAL  ● QUICK  ○ VEGAN

232
cals

★★★★★ *I made this last night for dinner and it was delicious! The sauce is so scrumptious and fairly easy to make. My family loved it, too! Highly recommend!* **CTILTON**

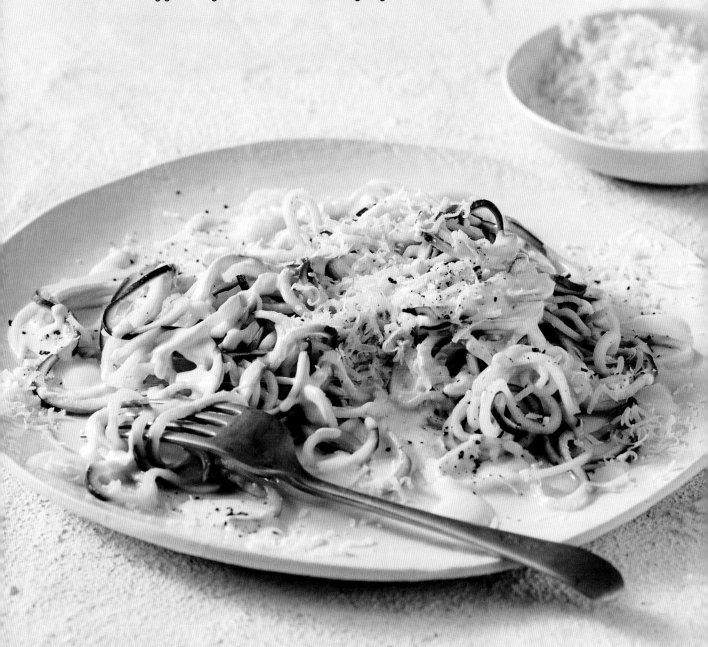

# MISO ROASTED
# EGGPLANT

Turn eggplant into something spectacular with an easy miso glaze. The sprinkling of mico herbs makes this dish look as pretty as a picture.

**SERVES** 4 **PREP** 10 mins **COOK** 35 mins

2 eggplant, halved lengthways
100g (⅓ cup) miso paste
2 tbs mirin
1 tbs cooking sake
1 tbs caster sugar
Toasted sesame seeds and fresh
  micro herbs, to serve

**1** Preheat oven to 200°C/180°C fan forced. Heat a non-stick frying pan over medium heat. Score the eggplant flesh deeply in a diamond pattern without cutting through the skin. Brush with olive oil. Cook, cut-side down, in the pan for 3 minutes or until golden.

**2** Transfer to a baking tray, cut-side up. Combine the miso paste, mirin, sake and caster sugar in a small bowl. Brush mixture over the cut-side of the eggplant. Roast for 30 minutes or until tender.

**3** Transfer miso eggplant to a serving plate and drizzle over any cooking juices. Sprinkle with sesame seeds and micro herbs, to serve.

**COOK'S NOTE**

Serve with some steamed rice and a salad for a light, but satisfying, meal.

## NUTRITION (PER SERVE)

| CALS | FAT | SAT FAT | PROTEIN | CARBS |
|------|-----|---------|---------|-------|
| 307 | 24g | 13.6g | 5.8g | 38.9g |

★★★★★

*The top caramelised and the skin was soft enough to eat. Great flavour combination.* **AMY LEECH 86**

● EASY  ○ FAMILY-FRIENDLY  ● GLUTEN FREE  ● LOW CAL  ○ QUICK  ○ VEGAN

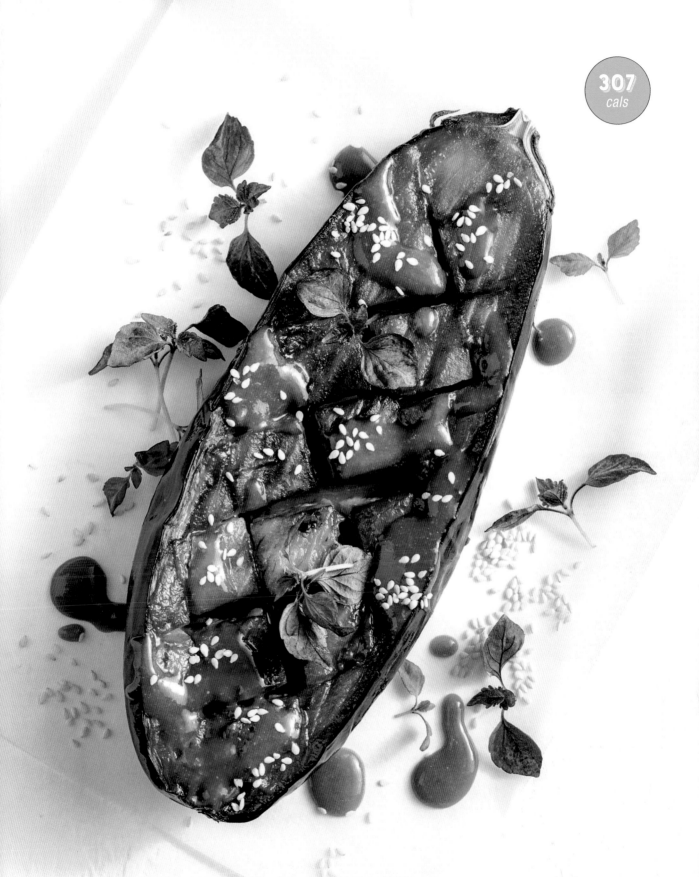

307
cals

# QUICK THAI TOFU NOODLE SALAD

For a quick and easy vegan main, try this flavoursome Thai noodle salad, tossed with soft tofu, fresh herbs and fresh seasonal vegetables.

**SERVES** 4  **PREP** 10 mins  **COOK** 15 mins

200g thin flat rice noodles
2 tsp sesame oil
80g tube Thai stir-in seasoning paste
400g silken tofu (see note)
½ cup fresh Thai basil leaves, plus extra, to serve
½ cup fresh coriander leaves
2 carrots, peeled, shredded
1 small red onion, very thinly sliced
2 tsp soy sauce
2 limes, 1 juiced, 1 cut into wedges
1 cup bean sprouts
1 corncob, kernels removed
Maple flavoured cashews, chopped, to serve (optional)
Fresh red chilli, chopped, to serve

1 Place noodles in a large heatproof bowl. Cover with boiling water. Set aside for 10 minutes or until softened. Drain and refresh under cold running water.

2 Heat sesame oil in a non-stick frying pan over medium heat. Add seasoning paste and cook for 30 seconds. Add tofu and cook, stirring, for 3-4 minutes until 'scrambled' and lightly browned. Remove from heat. Stir through basil and half the coriander.

3 Combine noodles, carrot, onion and remaining coriander in a large bowl. Drizzle with the soy and lime juice. Toss to combine.

4 Arrange noodle salad on a serving platter. Top with tofu, bean sprouts and corn. Scatter with cashew, chilli and extra basil. Serve with lime wedges.

**COOK'S NOTE**

Choose a soft tofu so it breaks up while it cooks and resembles scrambled egg.

## NUTRITION (PER SERVE)

| CALS | FAT | SAT FAT | PROTEIN | CARBS |
|------|-----|---------|---------|-------|
| 372 | 8g | 1g | 13g | 55g |

○ EASY   ○ FAMILY-FRIENDLY   ● GLUTEN FREE   ● LOW CAL   ● QUICK   ● VEGAN

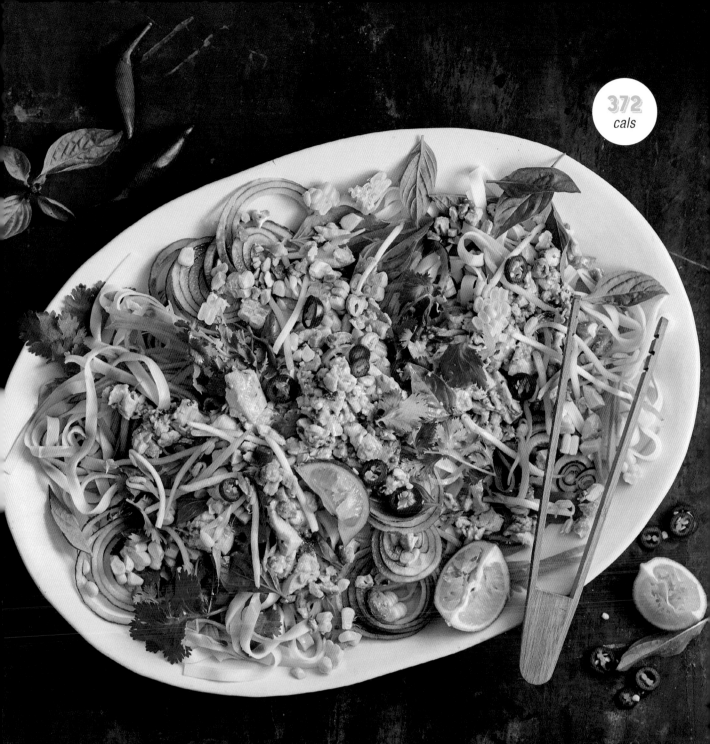

372 cals

★★★★★

*This salad was so easy to prepare, and very tasty; a nice change from the traditional salads and something the whole family enjoyed, including the children. I used maple flavoured cashews which were optional, however they did add that extra twist.* **TIGERS2018**

# SPICY TOMATO BLACK BEAN BOWL

Black beans are chock-full of antioxidants, fibre and protein. With added spices, tomato, sweet potato, egg and avo, you have a bowlful of yum!

**SERVES** 4  **PREP** 15 mins  **COOK** 30 mins

500g sweet potato, peeled, cut into 2cm pieces
1 tsp olive oil
1 red onion, finely chopped
2 garlic cloves, crushed
1 tsp paprika
1 tsp ground cumin
2 large vine-ripened tomatoes, chopped
400g can black beans, rinsed, drained
4 eggs
100g baby rocket
½ ripe avocado, coarsely mashed
2 tsp hot chilli sauce, to drizzle

1 Preheat oven to 200°C/180°C fan forced. Line a baking tray with baking paper. Place sweet potato on the prepared tray and spray lightly with oil. Bake for 25 minutes or until golden and tender.

2 Meanwhile, heat the oil in a large non-stick frying pan over medium heat. Add the onion and cook, stirring, for 5 minutes or until softened. Add the garlic, paprika and cumin. Cook, stirring, for 1 minute or until aromatic. Add the tomato and black beans. Cook for 5 minutes or until tomato is softened. Season. Roughly mash beans with a fork.

3 Lightly spray a clean, large non-stick frying pan with oil. Heat over medium-high heat. Fry eggs for 3-4 minutes or until cooked to your liking. Remove from the heat.

4 Divide the bean mixture, sweet potato and rocket among 4 serving bowls. Top each with a fried egg, avocado, cracked black pepper and a drizzle of chilli sauce. Serve.

**COOK'S NOTE**

Complete step 2 only, and place bean mixture on bed of corn chips. Top with grated cheddar, sour cream and avo for a tasty nachos.

## NUTRITION (PER SERVE)

| CALS | FAT | SAT FAT | PROTEIN | CARBS |
|------|-----|---------|---------|-------|
| 309 | 12g | 3g | 15g | 29g |

● EASY  ● FAMILY-FRIENDLY  ● GLUTEN FREE  ● LOW CAL  ○ QUICK  ○ VEGAN

309
cals

★ ★ ★ ★ ★
*Replaced the rocket with roasted broccoli and added couscous. Will make again.* **SKYFORGER**

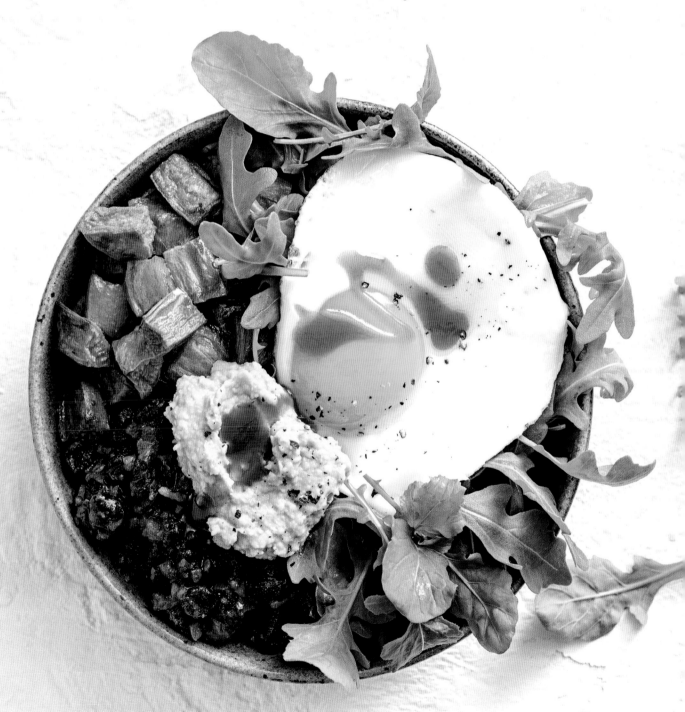

# MEXICAN ZUCCHINI SLICE

A delicious Mexican-inspired vegie slice that can be easily made ahead to spice up a busy weekday evening or take to work for lunch.

**SERVES** 4   **PREP** 5 mins   **COOK** 25 mins

5 eggs
3 egg whites
3 tsp Mexican spice mix
2 zucchini, grated
1 large carrot, grated
4 green shallots, thinly sliced
80g (½ cup) frozen peas, thawed
40g (¼ cup) self-raising flour
½ cup chopped fresh coriander
   leaves, plus extra leaves, to serve
60g cheddar, coarsely grated
1 avocado, sliced
1 tomato, cut into wedges
Sriracha, to drizzle

1. Preheat oven to 200°C/180°C fan forced. Grease a 26cm ovenproof frying pan with oil.

2. Whisk the eggs and egg whites in a large bowl until combined. Add spice mix and season well. Add zucchini, carrot, shallot and peas. Stir to combine. Add flour, coriander and half the cheese. Stir until combined.

3. Pour mixture into prepared pan and sprinkle with the remaining cheese. Bake for 20-25 minutes or until golden and cooked through.

4. Top with avocado, tomato and extra coriander. Drizzle with sriracha, to serve.

**COOK'S NOTE**

Make this slice up to 2 days ahead. Keep covered in the fridge, then gently warm in the oven before adding the fresh toppings, to serve.

## NUTRITION (PER SERVE)

| CALS | FAT | SAT FAT | PROTEIN | CARBS |
|------|-----|---------|---------|-------|
| 339 | 20g | 7g | 20g | 16g |

○ EASY   ● FAMILY-FRIENDLY   ○ GLUTEN FREE   ● LOW CAL   ● QUICK   ○ VEGAN

339
cals

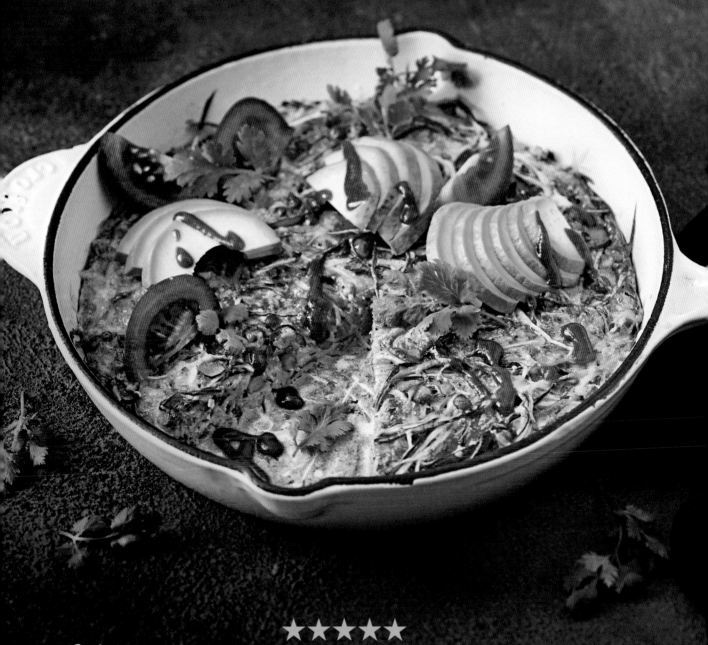

★★★★★

*We made this on the weekend and added some fresh asparagus, as we had some on hand. A very tasty and easy-to-make dish. It was just as tasty the next day. Loved it.* SG666

# BEETROOT VEGIE BURGERS

Fresh grated beetroot is high in folate and gives these vegie burgers great colour and taste. Prep ahead and you have a quick and easy midweek meal.

**SERVES** 4  **PREP** 15mins (+ cooling)  **COOK** 20 mins

1½ tbs extra virgin olive oil
1 small brown onion, finely chopped
1 carrot, peeled, coarsely grated
1 small beetroot, peeled,
    coarsely grated
2 tsp korma curry paste
750g can four bean mix,
    rinsed, drained
½ cup fresh coriander leaves
20g (¼ cup) quinoa flakes,
    plus extra 2 tbs
2 wholegrain (or sourdough) rolls,
    split, toasted
80ml (⅓ cup) beetroot tzatziki
Baby spinach leaves, to serve
1 Lebanese cucumber, sliced
    into ribbons
Micro herbs, to serve (optional)

1 Heat 2 tsp oil in a non-stick frying pan over medium heat. Add the onion and cook, stirring, for 5 minutes or until softened. Add the carrot and beetroot. Cook, stirring, for 2 minutes. Add the curry paste and cook, stirring, for 1 minute or until aromatic. Transfer to a large bowl and set aside to cool completely.

2 Add the bean mix and coriander to a food processor and process until coarsely chopped. Add to the onion mixture with the quinoa. Use clean hands to mix until well combined. Shape mixture into 4 flat patties. Place extra quinoa on a plate. Press patties into quinoa to lightly coat.

3 Heat the remaining oil in a large frying pan over medium-high heat. Add the patties and cook for 3-4 minutes each side or until golden. Transfer to paper towel to drain.

4 Top roll bases with tzatziki, spinach, beetroot patties, cucumber and herbs. Place roll tops and serve.

## COOK'S NOTE

Get ahead. Complete steps 1 and 2 on a weekend, then keep patties in an airtight container in the fridge (separated with plastic wrap) for up to 3 days. Continue from step 3 to cook and serve your busy weeknight meal.

## NUTRITION (PER SERVE)

| CALS | FAT | SAT FAT | PROTEIN | CARBS |
|------|-----|---------|---------|-------|
| 378 | 12g | 2g | 16g | 45g |

● EASY  ● FAMILY-FRIENDLY  ○ GLUTEN FREE  ● LOW CAL  ○ QUICK  ○ VEGAN

★★★★★ *These burgers are extremely tasty. Very quick & easy to make. Love them.* **SHOGUNRETRIEVE**

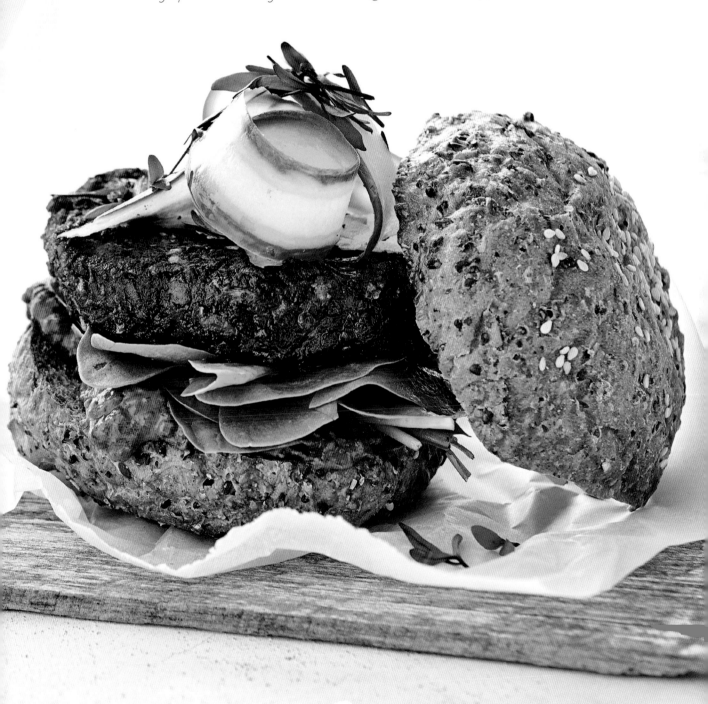

# MUFFIN PAN
# FRITTATAS

This cheesy vegetarian frittatas contain five different types of roasted vegetables for a delicious lunch you can make ahead.

**SERVES** 6 **PREP** 15 mins **COOK** 1 hour

- 1 (about 400g) sweet potato, cut into 2cm pieces
- 2 (about 250g) lebanese (slender) eggplants, coarsely chopped
- 1 small red onion, cut into wedges
- 1 small red capsicum, deseeded, cut into thick strips
- 1 zucchini, halved lengthways, coarsely chopped
- 1 tbs olive oil
- 6 eggs
- 2 tsp chopped fresh continental parsley leaves
- 60g feta, crumbled

**1** Line 6 holes of a 185ml (¾ cup) Texas muffin pan with baking paper, allowing the paper to overhang the sides.

**2** Preheat oven to 200°C/180°C fan forced. Grease 2 large baking trays. Line with baking paper. Spread the sweet potato, eggplant, onion, capsicum and zucchini over prepared trays. Drizzle over the oil and season. Bake for 30 minutes or until tender. Set aside on trays to cool.

**3** Heat the oven to 180°C/160°C fan forced. Whisk the eggs in a small bowl. Add the parsley and season. Toss the roasted vegetables together then divide between prepared muffin pan holes. Carefully pour the egg mixture over the top then sprinkle with the feta. Bake for 30 minutes or until just set. Serve.

**COOK'S NOTE**

This is a great recipe to use up any leftover roasted vegies (or cook extra if you have the oven on anyway). You'll need about 4 cups of chopped roasted veg.

## NUTRITION (PER SERVE)

| CALS | FAT | SAT FAT | PROTEIN | CARBS |
|------|-----|---------|---------|-------|
| 198 | 10.1g | 3.2g | 11.2g | 13.6g |

★★★★★ *I just love roasted vegetables, and to have them in a muffin was supee satisfying. Thanks for the recipe.* **MURRAYMINT**

● EASY ● FAMILY-FRIENDLY ○ GLUTEN FREE ● LOW CAL ○ QUICK ○ VEGAN

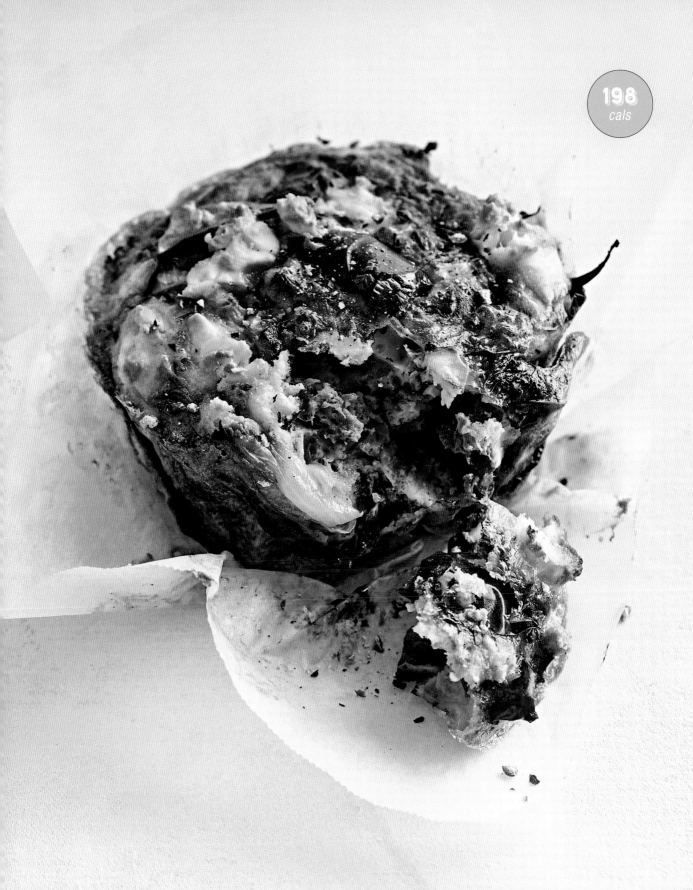

# CREAMY TOMATO SOUP WITH RAVIOLI

Our easy, creamy vegie-filled vegan soup is made all the more tempting loaded up with vegan spinach and ricotta ravioli.

**SERVES** 4 **PREP** 10 mins **COOK** 30 mins

1 tbs extra virgin olive oil, plus extra, to serve
1 brown onion, chopped
2 garlic cloves, chopped
800g can whole peeled tomatoes
1 large potato, peeled, diced
500ml (2 cups) vegetable stock
1 tsp dried oregano
300g pkt vegan spinach and ricotta ravioli
250ml (1 cup) almond milk
150g baby spinach, plus extra, to serve
Fresh basil leaves, to serve

**1** Heat the oil in a large saucepan over medium-high heat. Add the onion and garlic. Season. Cook, stirring occasionally, for 6 minutes or until onion is softened. Add the tomato, potato, vegie stock and oregano. Bring to the boil. Cover, reduce heat to medium and simmer for 20 minutes. Remove from heat.

**2** Meanwhile, cook the pasta following packet directions. Drain well.

**3** Pour the almond milk into the soup mixture. Using a stick blender, blend until smooth. Add spinach and stir until starting to wilt. Divide soup and pasta among serving bowls. Season with pepper. Drizzle with a little extra oil. Serve topped with basil leaves and extra spinach.

**COOK'S NOTE**

Even without the pasta this soup makes a satisfying meal with some crusty bread for dipping.

## NUTRITION (PER SERVE)

| CALS | FAT | SAT FAT | PROTEIN | CARBS |
|------|-----|---------|---------|-------|
| 319 | 8.6g | 1.3g | 8.5g | 46.9g |

★★★★★ *This was a welcome change to the usual pasta and sauce. As soon as I saw a vegan spinach and ricotta ravioli, I knew this would be a new family favourite!* **TRACEY1901**

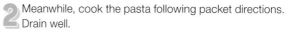

○ EASY  ● FAMILY-FRIENDLY  ○ GLUTEN FREE  ● LOW CAL  ○ QUICK  ● VEGAN

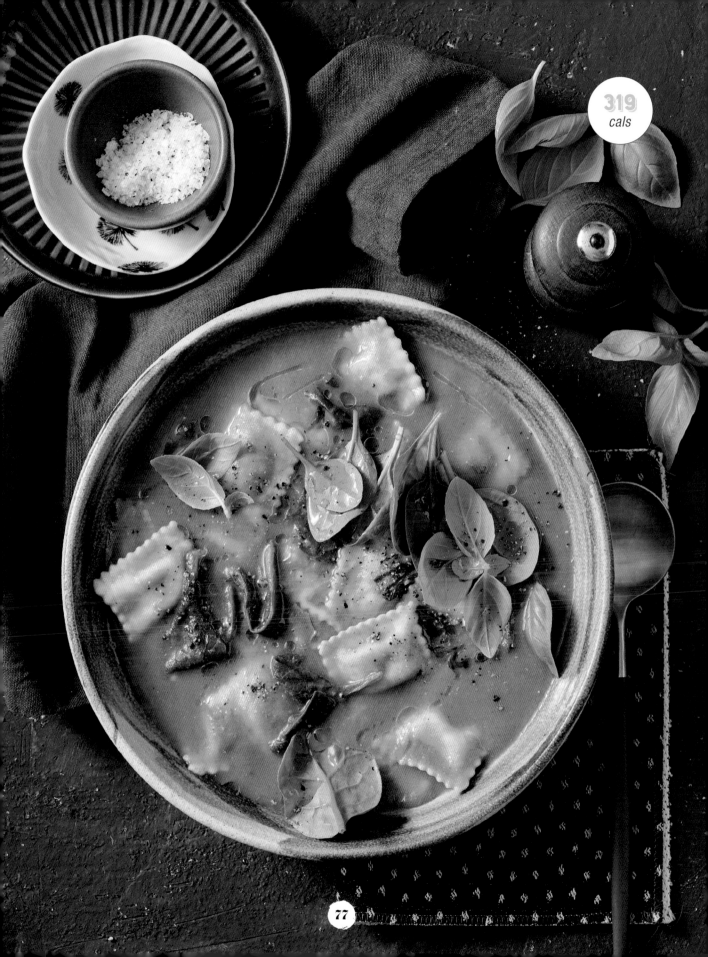

319 cals

# SPINACH & MUSHIE MINI QUICHES

These easy, savoury little quiches are great for a party, kids' lunch boxes or even a make-ahead brekky on the go. Eat them warm or not – it's up to you.

**MAKES** 12  **PREP** 15 mins  **COOK** 35 mins

3 sheets frozen shortcrust pastry, just thawed
1 tbs olive oil
1 small brown onion, finely chopped
200g Swiss brown mushrooms, thickly sliced
120g pkt baby spinach
55g (1 cup) finely grated gruyere or cheddar
5 eggs
300ml ctn pouring cream

**1** Preheat oven to 180°C/160°C fan forced. Lightly grease two 6-hole 125ml (½ cup) muffin pans.

**2** Use a 12cm-diameter round pastry cutter to cut 4 discs from each pastry sheet. Push the discs into the muffin pan holes, gently pressing any creases in the pastry so that it lies flat, and easing the pastry up the side of each hole to reach the top of the pan.

**3** Line the pastry cases with baking paper and fill with pastry weights or rice. Bake for 15 minutes. Remove paper and weights or rice. Set aside for 10 minutes to cool slightly.

**4** Meanwhile, heat the oil in a large frying pan over medium heat. Add the onion. Cook, stirring, for 5 minutes or until softened. Add the mushroom. Cook, stirring occasionally, for 3-4 minutes or until softened. Add the spinach and stir until wilted. Transfer mixture to a plate and set aside to cool slightly.

**5** Divide half the cheese among the pastry cases. Top with the mushroom mixture, reserving a few tablespoons. Sprinkle with remaining cheese and reserved mushroom mixture. Whisk the eggs and cream in a jug until well combined. Carefully pour egg mixture into the pastry cases, filling to the top edge of the pastry. Bake for 20 minutes or until just set and lightly browned.

## NUTRITION (PER SERVE)

| CALS | FAT | SAT FAT | PROTEIN | CARBS |
|------|-----|---------|---------|-------|
| 304 | 23.1g | 11.5g | 1.2g | 7.2g |

○ EASY  ● FAMILY-FRIENDLY  ○ GLUTEN FREE  ● LOW CAL  ○ QUICK  ○ VEGAN

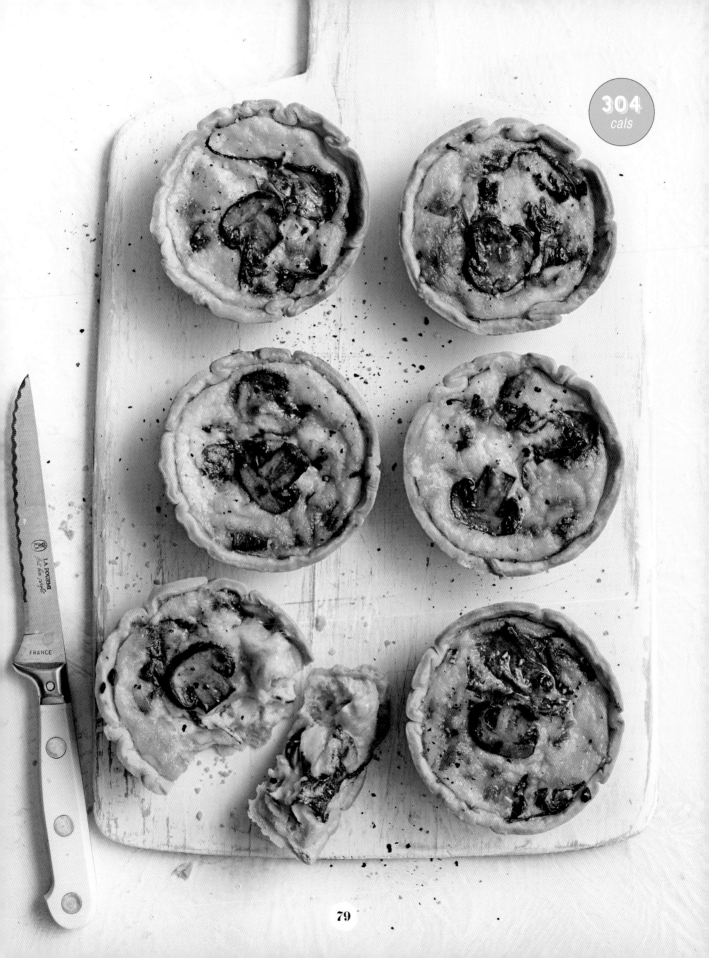

304
cals

# STICKY TOFU FRIED RICE

Toss together this saucy weeknight meal! It's low-calorie, dotted with ginger and garlic tofu, and the sauce is so delectably sticky, you'll want seconds.

**SERVES** 4  **PREP** 10 mins  **COOK** 10 mins

2 tbs light soy sauce
2 tbs honey
1 tbs Chinese rice wine
1 tsp sambal oelek
2 tsp rice bran oil
1 tbs shredded fresh ginger
2 garlic cloves, finely chopped
375g pkt firm tofu, cut into
   1cm pieces
2 zucchinis, trimmed, halved
   lengthways, sliced
250g pkt microwave brown rice
   and quinoa
200g frozen edamame, blanched,
   podded
1 cup fresh basil leaves
Shredded green shallot, to serve

**1** Combine soy sauce, honey, rice wine and sambal oelek in a small jug with 2 tbs water. Set aside until required.

**2** Heat the oil in a wok over high heat. Add the ginger and garlic. Cook, stirring, for 30 seconds or until aromatic. Add the tofu and cook, gently stirring, being careful not to break up the tofu, for 2 minutes or until lightly browned.

**3** Add half the sauce mixture and cook, stirring often, for 5 minutes or until reduced and sticky. Add the zucchini and cook, stirring, for 1 minute or until lightly golden. Add the rice and quinoa mix, plus the remaining sauce. Stir to coat.

**4** Add edamame and cook, stirring, for 1 minute or until warmed through. Season with salt and white pepper. Toss through basil leaves and top with shallot, to serve.

## COOK'S NOTE

You'll find edamame in the freezer section of the supermarket, near the frozen peas and beans. Replace with 80g (½ cup) frozen peas, if you prefer.

## NUTRITION (PER SERVE)

| CALS | FAT | SAT FAT | PROTEIN | CARBS |
|------|-----|---------|---------|-------|
| 337 | 12g | 2g | 18g | 34g |

★★★★★ *This was a perfect balance of vegetables, rice/quinoa and tofu. The sticky honey and soy sauce coated everything wonderfully, so every spoonful was simply scrummy.* **SHAWNTHEPRAWN**

○ EASY  ○ FAMILY-FRIENDLY  ○ GLUTEN FREE  ● LOW CAL  ● QUICK  ○ VEGAN

337
cals

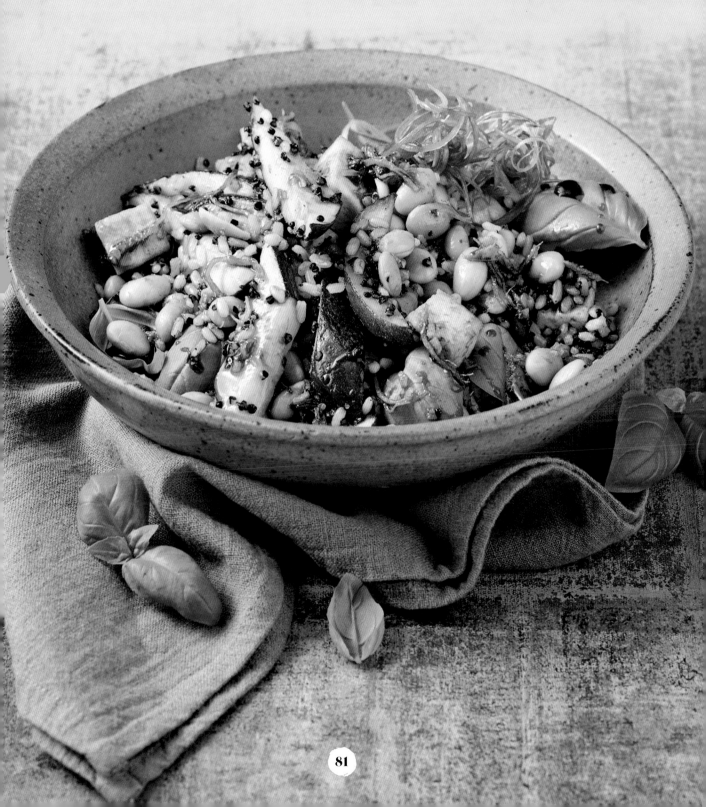

# SUPER EASY HALOUMI SALAD

Served up in just 20 minutes, this easy vego haloumi salad looks spectacular and makes the perfect light lunch or entertainer.

**SERVES** 6  **PREP** 10 mins  **COOK** 10 mins

250g pkt pearl couscous
2 x 250g pkts haloumi, sliced
1 tbs Moroccan spice mix
2 zucchini, sliced
250g punnet cherry tomato
   medley, halved
½ cup fresh continental
   parsley leaves
½ cup fresh mint leaves, torn
1 tbs tahini
2 tbs Greek yoghurt
1 small garlic clove, crushed
1 lemon, rind finely grated, juiced
2 tbs pomegranate arils
3 wholemeal pita breads,
   toasted, torn (optional)

**1** Cook couscous in a saucepan of boiling water following packet directions. Drain.

**2** Meanwhile, pat haloumi dry with paper towel. Sprinkle with spice mix. Spray a non-stick frying pan with oil and heat over medium heat. Cook haloumi for 1-2 minutes each side or until golden. Set aside. Spray pan with more oil. Cook zucchini for 1-2 minutes or until just coloured.

**3** Combine couscous, zucchini, tomato, parsley and mint in a large bowl. Season well. Combine tahini, yoghurt, garlic and lemon rind in a small bowl. Season. Stir in lemon juice.

**4** Arrange salad on a serving platter. Top with haloumi and pomegranate. Drizzle over dressing. Serve with pita.

**COOK'S NOTE**

Use it up: If you have leftover pomegranate arils, add to champagne with a dash of pomegranate or cranberry juice for a fruity cocktail.

## NUTRITION (PER SERVE)

| CALS | FAT | SAT FAT | PROTEIN | CARBS |
|------|------|---------|---------|-------|
| 376 | 16.6g | 9.8g | 21.5g | 13.2g |

★★★★★

*It's delicious. Only used half of the tahini as flavour is very strong.*

**KATRINACONSTANTIN**

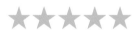

● EASY  ○ FAMILY-FRIENDLY  ● GLUTEN FREE  ● LOW CAL  ● QUICK  ○ VEGAN

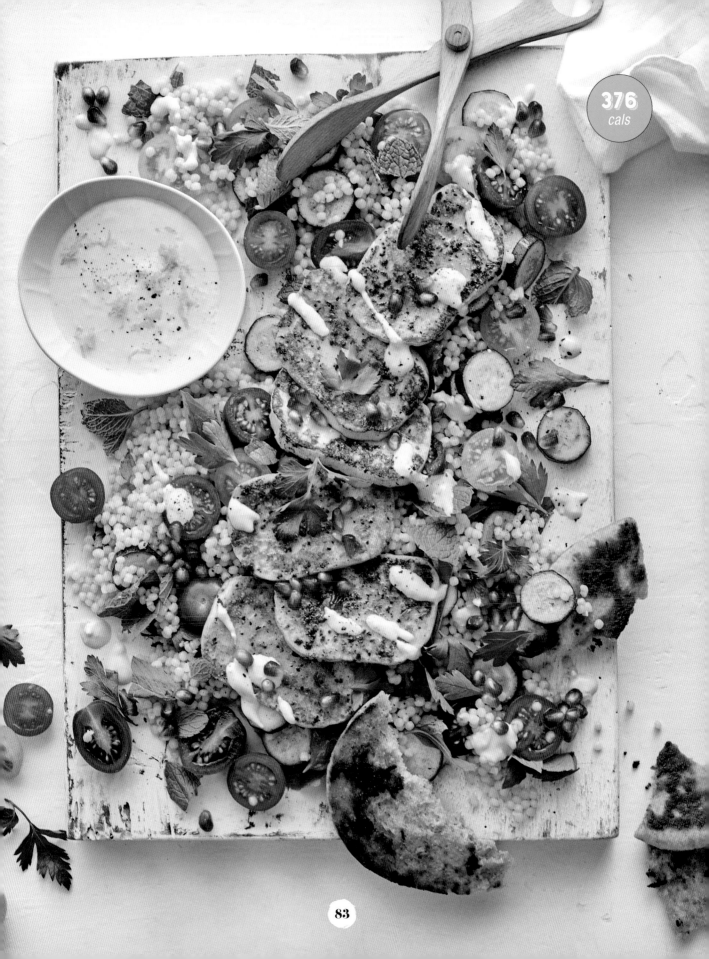

# CAULI RICE & KORMA TOFU GRILL

Healthy cauli rice is in demand right now, and so is our grilled Indian-spiced tofu. Put them together and you have a deliciously light dinner for four.

**SERVES** 4  **PREP** 15 mins (+ 15 mins marinating)  **COOK** 10 mins

2 tbs natural yoghurt
1 tbs korma curry paste
250g firm tofu, drained, cut into
    1cm-thick slices
1 small head (700g) cauliflower,
    cut into florets
2 tsp coconut oil
1 red onion, finely chopped
3 garlic cloves, crushed
2 tsp finely grated fresh ginger
1 long fresh green chilli, finely
    chopped
400g can no-added-salt lentils,
    rinsed, drained
150g baby spinach
Fresh coriander leaves and lime
    wedges, to serve

1 Combine the yoghurt and curry paste in a shallow dish. Add the tofu and turn to coat. Cover with plastic wrap. Place in the fridge for 15 minutes to marinate.

2 Working in batches, process the cauliflower in a food processor until it resembles rice. Transfer to a bowl.

3 Heat the oil in a large wok over high heat. Add the onion and cook, stirring, for 2 minutes or until softened. Add the garlic, ginger and chilli. Cook, stirring, for 1 minute or until aromatic. Add the cauli rice and cook, stirring, for 2-3 minutes or until just tender. Add the lentils and spinach, and stir for 1 minute or until warmed through. Set aside and cover to keep warm.

4 Preheat a barbecue grill or chargrill pan on medium-high. Lift tofu from the marinade and lightly spray with oil. Cook for 2 minutes each side or until golden. Serve cauli rice mixture with the tofu, sprinkled with coriander and with lime wedges alongside.

**COOK'S NOTE**

For a cheesy twist, swap the tofu for 200g paneer, cut into 1cm-thick slices. Marinate as in step 1 and cook in a non-stick frying pan for 1-2 minutes each side.

## NUTRITION (PER SERVE)

| CALS | FAT | SAT FAT | PROTEIN | CARBS |
|------|-----|---------|---------|-------|
| 259 | 10g | 4g | 19g | 17g |

● EASY   ○ FAMILY-FRIENDLY   ● GLUTEN FREE   ● LOW CAL   ○ QUICK   ○ VEGAN

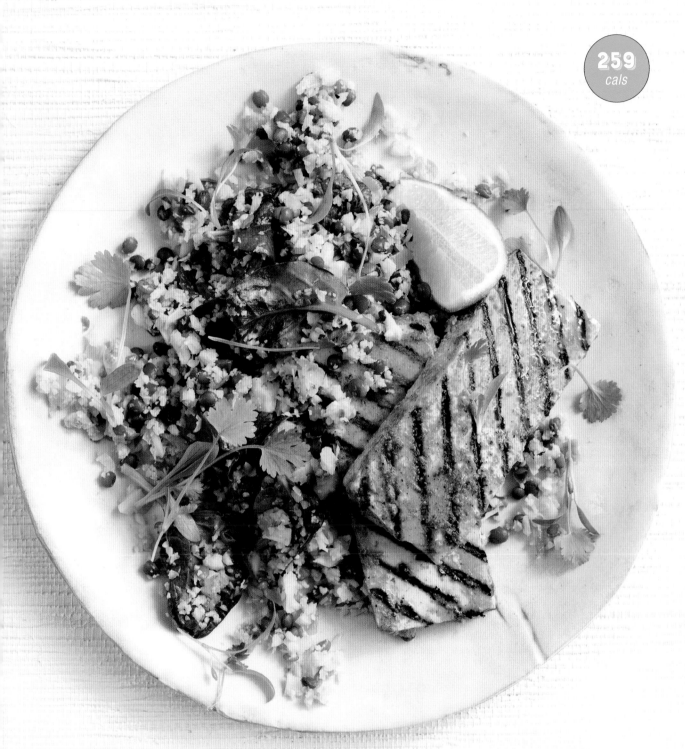

259 cals

★★★★★ *This was delicious and so easy. I used tandoori paste and chilli flakes instead of the korma and green chilli (because that is what I had). A healthy quick meal.* **JWILS466**

# JATZ CRACKER & SPINACH QUICHE

We took a popular cracker and crushed it to make the base. Then we added a creamy cheesy veg topping to make a new family favourite.

**SERVES** 12  **PREP** 25 mins (+ chilling & cooling)  **COOK** 40 mins

225g pkt Jatz crackers
150g butter, melted
2 tsp olive oil
2 garlic cloves, finely chopped
250g pkt frozen chopped spinach
250g pkt cream cheese, chopped,
   at room temperature
85g (⅓ cup) sour cream
80ml (⅓ cup) milk
3 eggs
2 green shallots, thinly sliced,
   plus extra, to serve
2 tbs chopped fresh mint
60g feta, crumbled
80g (1 cup) coarsely grated cheddar
Green salad, to serve (optional)

**1** Break up crackers into a food processor. Process until very finely crushed. Add the butter and pulse to combine. Press the mixture over the base and side of a 3cm deep, 23cm (base measurement) round fluted tart tin with removable base. Place in the fridge for 15 minutes to chill.

**2** Meanwhile, heat the oil in a frying pan over medium-high heat. Add the garlic and cook, stirring, for 1 minute or until aromatic. Add the spinach. Cook, stirring often, for 5 minutes or until spinach has defrosted and any excess liquid has evaporated. Set aside until required.

**3** Preheat oven to 180°C/160°C fan forced. Bake the quiche crust for 10 minutes or until golden. Set aside to cool slightly.

**4** While the crust is cooling, use electric beaters to beat the cream cheese until smooth. Beat in the sour cream and milk until combined. Add the eggs, 1 at a time, beating well after each addition. Stir in the spinach mixture, shallot and mint. Season.

**5** Pour the cream cheese mixture into the baked crust. Sprinkle with feta and cheddar. Bake for 20 minutes or until filling is set. Set aside to cool for 1 hour or until at room temperature. Sprinkle with extra green shallot, to serve.

## NUTRITION (PER SERVE)

| CALS | FAT | SAT FAT | PROTEIN | CARBS |
|------|-----|---------|---------|-------|
| 351 | 28.95g | 65.5g | 8.65g | 14.6g |

● EASY  ● FAMILY-FRIENDLY  ○ GLUTEN FREE  ● LOW CAL  ○ QUICK  ○ VEGAN

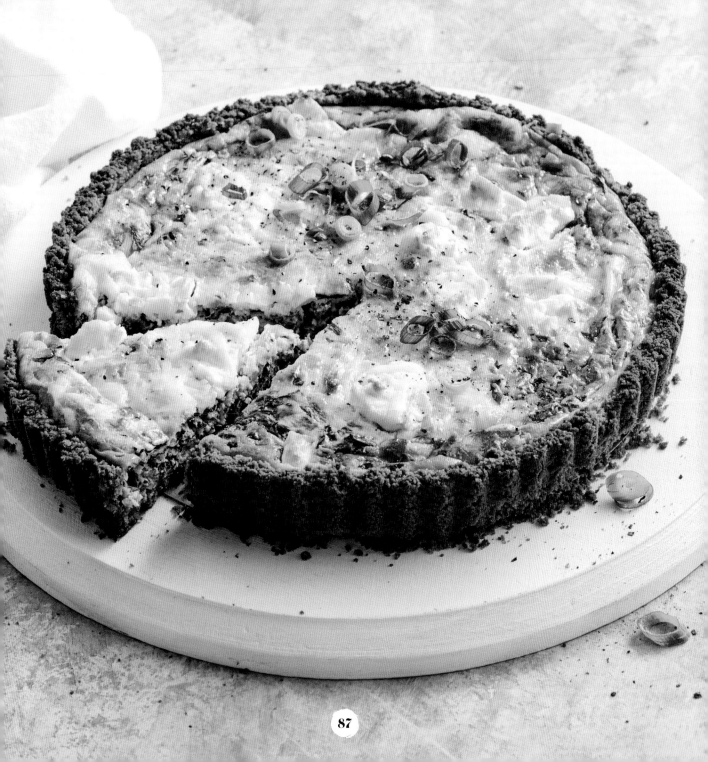

★★★★★
*Jatz are my favourite crackers and they worked perfectly for the base of this quiche. Great idea!* **CHARLIER**

351
cals

# CURRIED TOFU & VEGETABLE PATTIES

Go meat-free with these speedy patties that are delightfully crunchy on the outside and tender inside. They're ideal for dinner or a work lunch box.

**MAKES** 12  **PREP** 15 mins (+ cooling)  **COOK** 25 mins

¼ small cauliflower
1 tbs vegetable oil, plus extra, to shallow-fry
150g orange sweet potato, coarsely grated
½ red capsicum, finely chopped
55g (⅓ cup) frozen peas
2 green shallots, thinly sliced
2 tsp curry powder
250g firm tofu, coarsely grated
135g (1 cup) cold cooked brown rice (see note)
100g (⅔ cup) plain flour
2 eggs, lightly beaten
Fresh coriander sprigs, mixed salad leaves and reduced-fat Greek-style yoghurt, to serve

1 Place cauliflower in a food processor and pulse to coarse crumbs. Heat the oil in a large frying pan over high heat. Add cauliflower and sweet potato. Cook, stirring, for 2-3 minutes or until just tender. Add capsicum, peas, shallot and curry powder. Cook, stirring, for 1 minute. Remove from heat and set aside to cool.

2 Using clean hands, squeeze out any excess moisture from the tofu and place in a large bowl. Add cooled cauliflower mixture, rice, flour and egg. Season. Stir well to combine.

3 Pour enough extra oil into a large frying pan to just cover the base of the pan. Heat over medium-high heat. Working in batches, add ⅓ cup of tofu mixture to the pan for each patty. Cook for 2-3 minutes each side or until golden and cooked through. Transfer to a plate lined with paper towel to drain. Cover to keep warm. Sprinkle with the coriander, and serve with salad leaves and yoghurt.

**COOK'S NOTE**

To save time, you could use 1 cup of 90-second microwave brown rice. Don't heat the rice before adding in step 2.

## NUTRITION (PER SERVE)

| CALS | FAT | SAT FAT | PROTEIN | CARBS |
|------|-----|---------|---------|-------|
| 397 | 17g | 4g | 15.8g | 42.5g |

○ EASY  ● FAMILY-FRIENDLY  ○ GLUTEN FREE  ● LOW CAL  ○ QUICK  ○ VEGAN

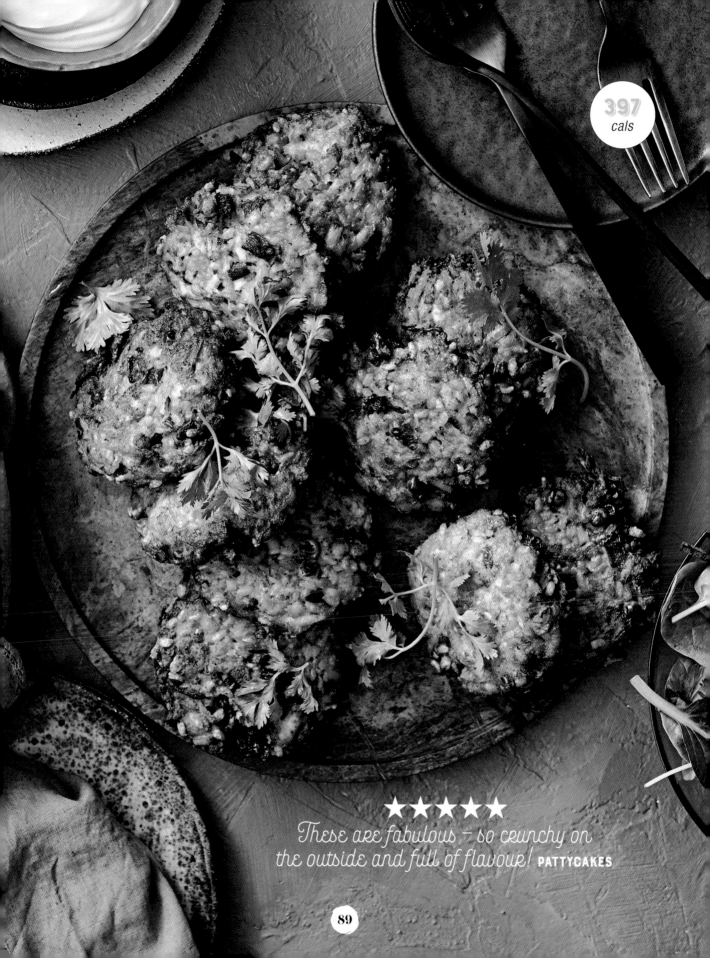

★ ★ ★ ★ ★

*These are fabulous – so crunchy on
the outside and full of flavour!* **PATTYCAKES**

397
*cals*

# HEALTHY MEXICAN FRIED RICE

Better than takeaway, our fried rice is packed with capsicum, corn and healthy black beans. Topped with tomato, avo and feta, you couldn't want for more!

**SERVES** 4  **PREP** 20 mins (+ 1 hour chilling)  **COOK** 35 mins

150g (¾ cup) brown rice
1 tbs olive oil
1 brown onion, chopped
1 red capsicum, deseeded, chopped
2 garlic cloves, crushed
2 tsp Mexican chilli powder
400g can black beans, rinsed,
    drained
300g can corn kernels, drained
2 tbs fresh lime juice
200g punnet grape tomatoes,
    chopped
¼ small red onion, finely chopped
1 small ripe firm avocado,
    quartered, sliced
125g feta, crumbled (optional)
Fresh coriander sprigs and
    lime halves, to serve

1 Cook the rice in a large saucepan of boiling water for 25 minutes or until tender. Drain well, spread over a large tray and place in the fridge, uncovered, for at least 1 hour.

2 Heat the oil in a large frying pan over medium heat. Add the brown onion and capsicum. Cook for 5 minutes or until softened. Add the garlic and chilli powder. Cook, stirring, for 30 seconds or until aromatic.

3 Add rice to the pan and cook, stirring, for 2 minutes until lightly fried and well combined with the onion mixture. Add the beans and corn. Cook, stirring often, until heated through. Pour in lime juice and toss to combine.

4 Combine the tomato and red onion in a bowl. Season. Divide rice mixture among serving bowls. Top with the tomato mixture, avocado, feta and coriander. Serve with the lime halves for squeezing over.

**COOK'S NOTE**

For a vegan meal, simply omit the feta, or use a plant-based cheese.

## NUTRITION (PER SERVE)

| CALS | FAT | SAT FAT | PROTEIN | CARBS |
|------|-----|---------|---------|-------|
| 372  | 11g | 1.5g    | 12.3g   | 46.5g |

★★★★★

*Yummy vegetarian meal. I used precooked brown and wild rice. I made guacamole for the top which was delicious.* **THEDOVELQUEEN**

● EASY  ● FAMILY-FRIENDLY  ● GLUTEN FREE  ● LOW CAL  ○ QUICK  ○ VEGAN

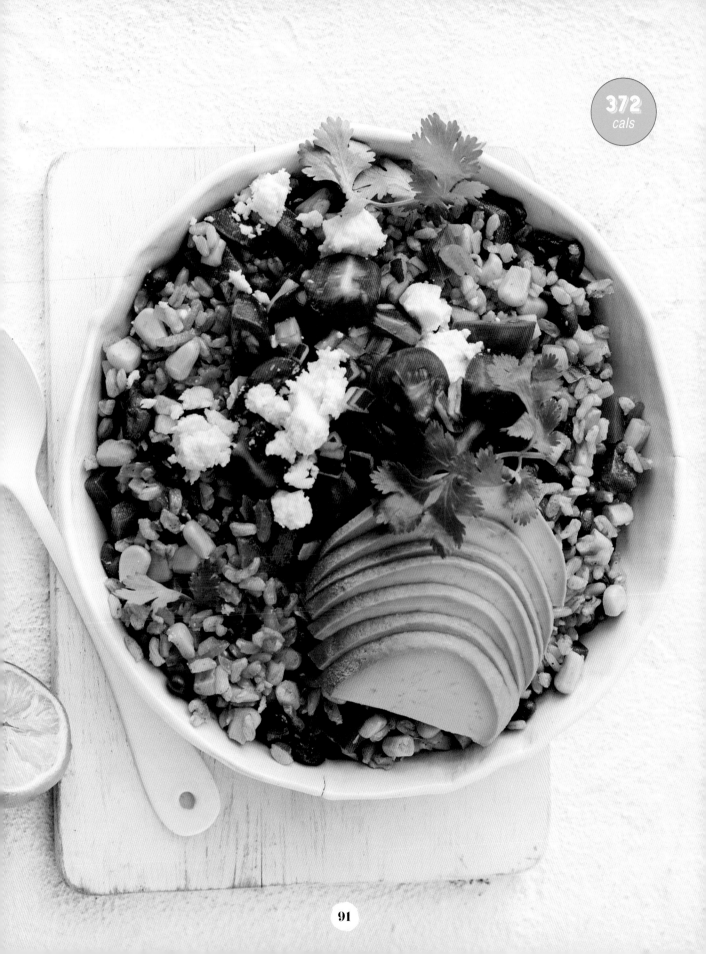

# ASPARAGUS FILO FRITTATAS

Fabulous hot or cold, you'll just love the way the flaky filo cases appear to dissolve in your mouth. You may need to make a double batch to go around!

**SERVES** 4 **PREP** 15 mins **COOK** 20 mins

4 sheets filo pastry, just thawed
1 bunch asparagus, trimmed, cut into 4cm lengths
1½ tbs finely chopped fresh chives
3 eggs
125ml (½ cup) milk
3 tsp chopped fresh thyme leaves
8 cherry truss tomatoes, separated, stems trimmed
80g mixed salad leaves, to serve

**1** Preheat oven to 180°C/160°C fan forced. Grease 4 holes of a 180ml (¾ cup) Texas muffin pan. Line each hole with strips of baking paper, with paper overhanging sides.

**2** Place 1 sheet of filo on a flat surface. Spray with oil. Place another sheet on top and spray with olive oil. Repeat layering with remaining 2 filo sheets, spraying each with oil.

**3** Cut filo stack into 4 even strips. Cut each strip in half to make 8 squares. Top 4 squares with the remaining 4 squares, rotating slightly to form a star shape. Gently press stacks into the prepared muffin pan holes.

**4** Divide asparagus and chives among filo cases. Whisk eggs, milk and thyme in a jug to combine. Season. Pour into filo cases to fill. Arrange 2 tomatoes on top of each filled case. Bake for 20 minutes or until filling is set and pastry is golden. Serve warm or at room temperature with salad leaves.

**COOK'S NOTE**

For a more substantial lunch crumble feta over the frittatas and serve with a side salad.

## NUTRITION (PER SERVE)

| CALS | FAT | SAT FAT | PROTEIN | CARBS |
|------|-----|---------|---------|-------|
| 145 | 6.6g | 2g | 8.3g | 11.1g |

★★★★★ *Super flaky, and I love the way the truss tomatoes burst as you bite into them.* **SHAWNTHEPRAWN**

● EASY ○ FAMILY-FRIENDLY ○ GLUTEN FREE ● LOW CAL ○ QUICK ○ VEGAN

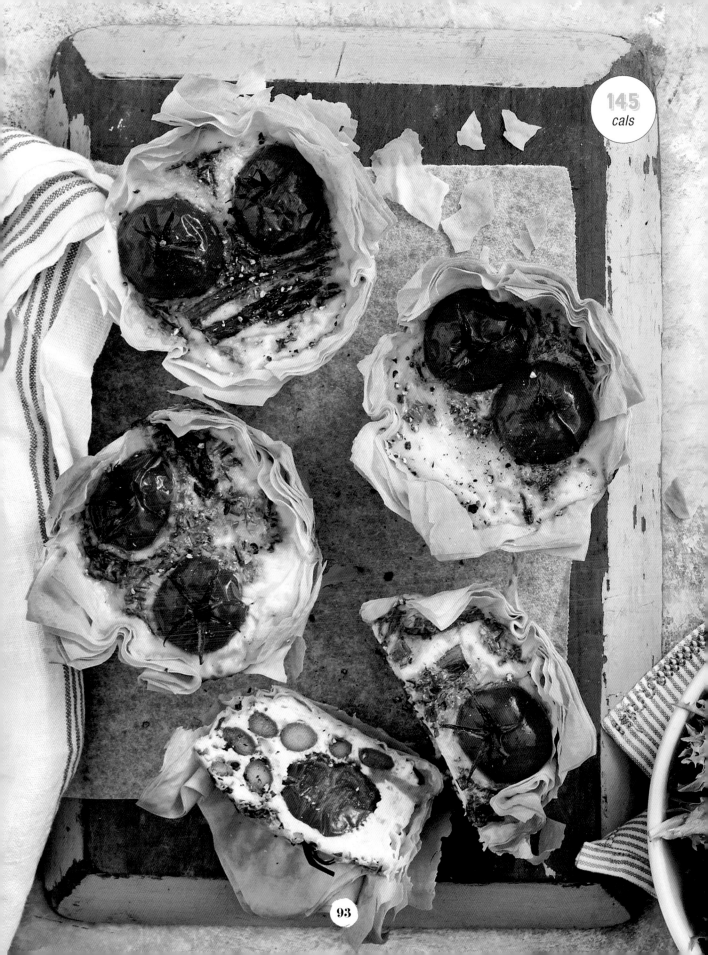

# SUNDAY SUPPER SOUFFLÉ

# OMELETTE

Lazy Sundays rule! Making the most of your leftover roast vegies,
this light-as-air soufflé omelette is a quick and easy end-of-week meal.

**SERVES** 2  **PREP** 10 mins  **COOK** 15 mins

1 tbs extra virgin olive oil
½ red onion or leek, thinly sliced
1 cup sliced mushrooms or zucchini
1 cup coarsely chopped kale
4 eggs, separated
40g (½ cup) coarsely grated cheddar
10g butter
1 cup leftover roasted vegetables
　(such as sweet potato, pumpkin
　and/or potato)
Finely grated parmesan,
　to serve (optional)

**1** Preheat oven to 220°C/200°C fan forced. Heat the oil in a non-stick ovenproof frying pan over medium-high heat. Add the onion and mushroom. Cook, stirring, for 3-4 minutes or until tender. Add the kale and cook, tossing, for 1-2 minutes until kale is slightly wilted. Transfer to a bowl. Wipe the pan clean.

**2** Whisk the egg whites until soft peaks form. Lightly fold in the yolks and one-third of the cheese.

**3** Heat the butter in the frying pan over medium-high heat. Add the egg mixture. Cook for 3-4 minutes or until the bottom is beginning to set. Sprinkle over mushroom mixture, roast vegetables and half the remaining cheese. Bake for 2-3 minutes or until vegetables are warm and the omelette is puffed and golden. Sprinkle remaining cheese over half the omelette. Carefully fold omelette in half. Sprinkle with parmesan to serve.

**COOK'S NOTE**

Instead of kale, you could use baby spinach or rocket, or a combination of all three!

## NUTRITION (PER SERVE)

| CALS | FAT | SAT FAT | PROTEIN | CARBS |
|------|-----|---------|---------|-------|
| 394 | 31.3g | 10.1g | 19g | 10.7g |

● EASY　● FAMILY-FRIENDLY　● GLUTEN FREE　● LOW CAL　● QUICK　○ VEGAN

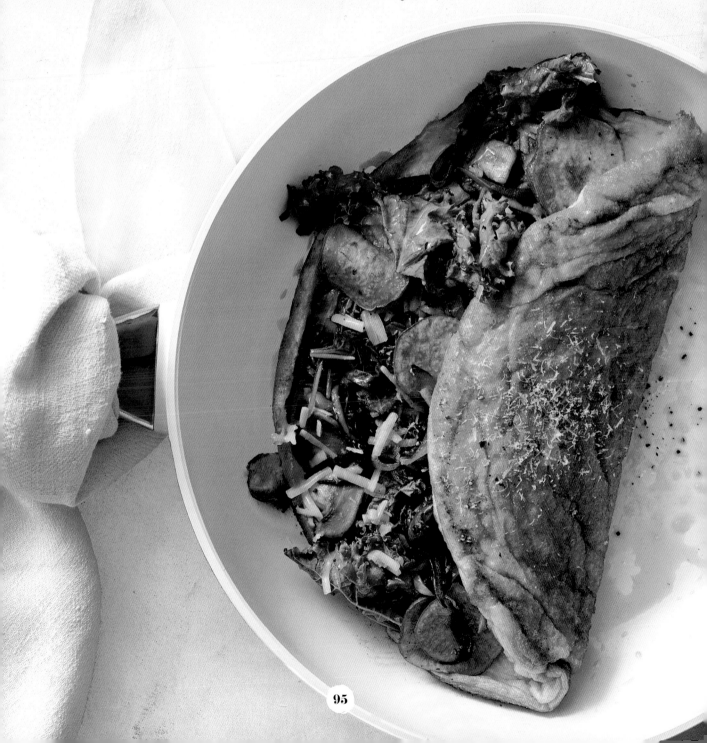

★ ★ ★ ★ ★

*This was fantastic. I used baby spinach, mushrooms and diced boiled veg. It was so light and very tasty. Even my husband who doesn't like omelettes commented on how good it was.* **GLENDA**

**394** cals

# FLAKY LENTIL & SILVERBEET PIES

Currants add a surprise sweetness to the silverbeet filling of these individual vego pies. And we just love the crunchy scrunchy filo top!

**SERVES** 4  **PREP** 20 mins  **COOK** 40 mins

2 tbs extra virgin olive oil
1 small brown onion, finely chopped
1 small carrot, peeled, finely chopped
2 tbs currants
1 garlic clove, crushed
1 bunch silverbeet, stems removed, leaves thinly sliced
2 tbs plain flour
310ml (1¼ cups) reduced-fat milk
400g can brown lentils, rinsed, drained
50g low-fat feta, crumbled
1 lemon, rind finely grated, juiced
4 sheets filo pastry
1 tsp chia seeds

1 Preheat oven to 190°C/170°C fan forced. Heat 1 tbs of oil in a non-stick frying pan over medium-low heat. Add the onion and carrot. Cook, stirring, for 3 minutes or until softened. Add the currants and garlic. Cook, stirring, for 2 minutes or until aromatic. Add silverbeet. Cover and cook, stirring occasionally, for 4 minutes or until silverbeet is just wilted. Increase heat to medium-high. Cook, stirring, for 2 minutes or until vegies are tender. Drain.

2 Heat remaining oil in a saucepan over medium-low heat. Add flour. Cook, stirring, for 1 minute or until foaming. Remove from heat. Slowly stir in milk until smooth. Reduce heat to low. Cook, stirring, for 4 minutes or until thickened.

3 Use hands to squeeze excess moisture from the silverbeet. Add silverbeet mixture to the milk mixture with the lentils, feta, lemon rind and 2 tbs lemon juice. Season. Stir to combine. Divide mixture among 4 greased 250ml (1 cup) ovenproof dishes.

4 Gently scrunch each filo sheet. Arrange on pies. Place dishes on a baking tray. Spray with olive oil. Sprinkle with chia seeds. Bake for 15-20 minutes or until golden. Serve.

## COOK'S NOTE

Swap the carrot for 2-3 large flat mushrooms, chopped, if you like, and omit the currants.

## NUTRITION (PER SERVE)

| CALS | FAT | SAT FAT | PROTEIN | CARBS |
| --- | --- | --- | --- | --- |
| 300 | 13g | 3g | 14g | 29g |

○ EASY   ● FAMILY-FRIENDLY   ○ GLUTEN FREE   ● LOW CAL   ○ QUICK   ○ VEGAN

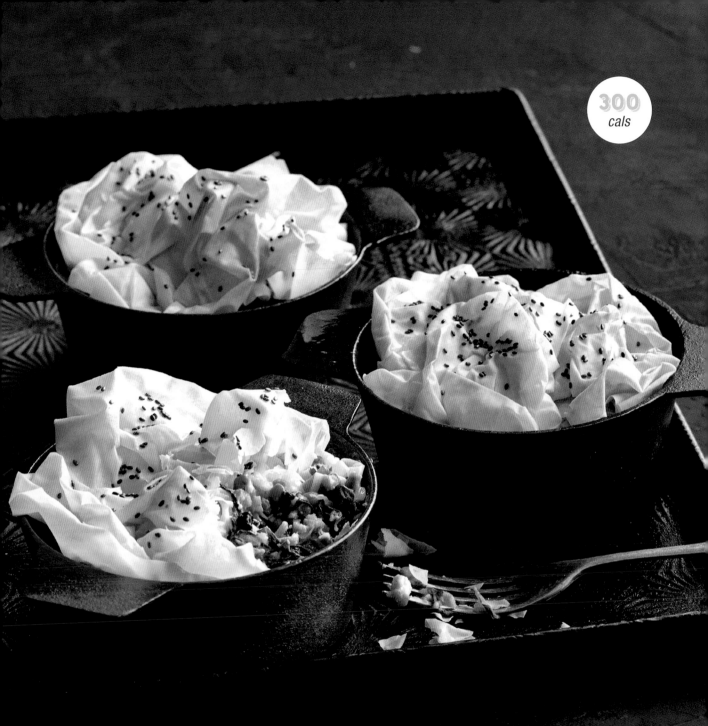

★★★★★

*This is such a delicious dish and not too difficult or time-consuming for the end product. Even my two-year-old loved it.* SARAH

# PUMPKIN CRUSTLESS QUICHE

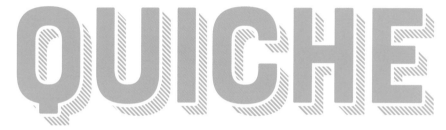

We've left the crust off altogether in this low-cal, gluten-free quiche that's loaded up with protein and a stack of all your favourite vegies.

**SERVES** 4 **PREP** 15 mins **COOK** 55 mins

500g pumpkin, peeled, deseeded, cut into 1cm-thick wedges

1 large red capsicum, deseeded, cut into 1.5cm pieces

2 tsp extra virgin olive oil

2 red onions, thinly sliced

2 garlic cloves, thinly sliced

2 tsp red wine vinegar

120g baby spinach

8 eggs

60ml (¼ cup) milk

60g Danish-style feta, crumbled

¼ cup chopped fresh basil leaves, plus extra leaves, to serve

1 tbs pine nuts, toasted

1 Preheat oven to 200°C/180°C fan forced. Line a large baking tray with baking paper. Arrange the pumpkin and capsicum on the prepared tray. Lightly spray with olive oil. Roast for 25 minutes or until golden and tender. Set aside to cool.

2 Meanwhile, heat the oil in a large non-stick frying pan over medium-low heat. Add the onion and cook, stirring often, for 10 minutes or until starting to caramelise. Add the garlic and vinegar. Cook, stirring often, for 5 minutes or until onion is light golden.

3 Place the spinach in a large heatproof bowl. Cover with boiling water and set aside for 10 seconds. Drain spinach and refresh under cold running water. When cool enough to handle, use hands to squeeze out excess water and chop.

4 Whisk the eggs and milk in a large bowl. Stir in the feta, basil and chopped spinach. Season.

5 Reduce oven to 180°C/160°C fan forced. Lightly grease a 16 x 26cm slice pan and line the base and sides with baking paper, allowing the paper to overhang the long sides. Arrange the roast vegetables and onion over the base of prepared pan. Evenly pour the egg mixture over the top. Bake for 30 minutes or until the quiche is puffed and golden. Turn onto a wire rack and leave for 10 minutes to cool slightly. Sprinkle with pine nuts. Serve sprinkled with extra basil leaves.

## NUTRITION (PER SERVE)

| CALS | FAT | SAT FAT | PROTEIN | CARBS |
|------|-----|---------|---------|-------|
| 326 | 20g | 5.7g | 20.7g | 12.5g |

○ EASY  ● FAMILY-FRIENDLY  ● GLUTEN FREE  ● LOW CAL  ○ QUICK  ○ VEGAN

326 cals

★★★★★
*Best dish ever!!!!! It was absolutely delicious!!!!!* **JULZRULZ**

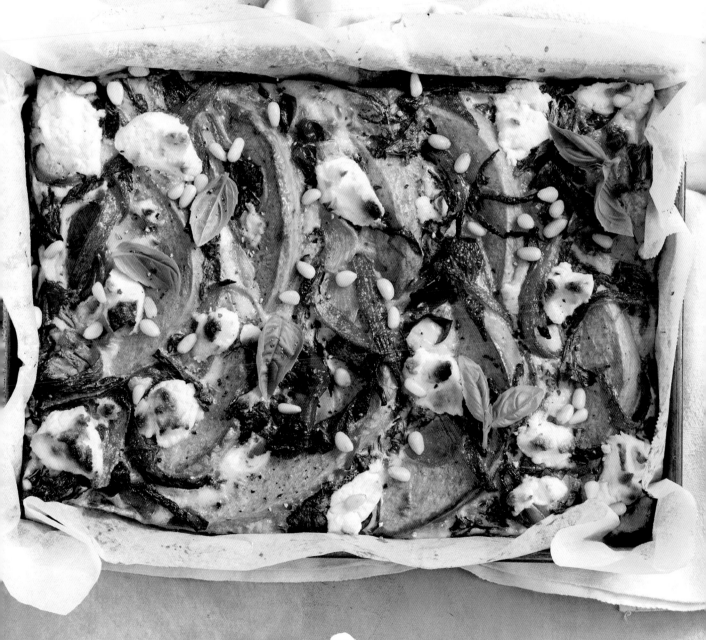

# SPINACH & FETA PULL-APART PIE

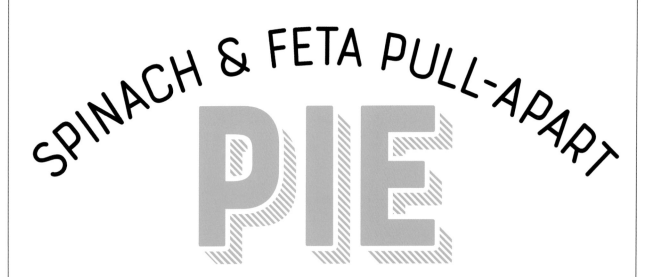

Stick it in the oven and that's dinner done. Each swirl is a delicious serving of crunchy filo and cheesy spinach filling. Watch them disappear!

**SERVES** 7 **PREP** 20 mins (+ cooling) **COOK** 35 mins

2 tbs olive oil
4 green shallots, thinly sliced
2 garlic cloves, crushed
280g packet baby spinach, coarsely chopped
200g creamy feta, crumbled
200g fresh ricotta
2 eggs, lightly beaten
¼ cup chopped fresh dill
14 sheets filo pastry, just thawed
100g butter, melted, cooled
Lemon wedges, to serve

1 Preheat oven to 200°C/180°C fan forced. Heat the oil in a 25cm (base measurement) ovenproof frying pan over medium heat. Add the shallot and garlic. Cook, stirring often, for 2 minutes or until softened. Transfer to a large bowl. Add the spinach to the pan, in batches, and cook, stirring, for 1 minute until wilted. Transfer to the bowl. Set aside to cool. Wipe the pan clean and lightly spray with olive oil.

2 Add the feta, ricotta, egg and dill to the cooled spinach mixture. Stir to combine. Season with black pepper.

3 Place pastry sheets on a clean work surface. Cover with a clean, dry tea towel, then a damp tea towel. Remove 1 sheet and brush with melted butter. Top with another sheet and brush with melted butter. Divide spinach mixture into 7 portions. Spread 1 portion along 1 long edge of pastry stack. Roll up firmly to enclose the filling. Coil into a snail shape and arrange, seam-side down in greased pan. Cover loosely with plastic wrap. Repeat with the remaining pastry sheets, butter and spinach mixture to make 6 more snail shapes, arranging snails with ends turned inward to keep their shape while cooking.

4 Brush snail tops with remaining butter and sprinkle with sea salt. Bake for 30 minutes or until the pastry is crisp and golden. Sprinkle with black pepper. Serve immediately with lemon wedges.

## NUTRITION (PER SERVE)

| CALS | FAT | SAT FAT | PROTEIN | CARBS |
|------|------|---------|---------|-------|
| 373 | 27.2g | 14.2g | 14.3g | 17.2g |

○ EASY   ● FAMILY-FRIENDLY   ○ GLUTEN FREE   ● LOW CAL   ○ QUICK   ○ VEGAN

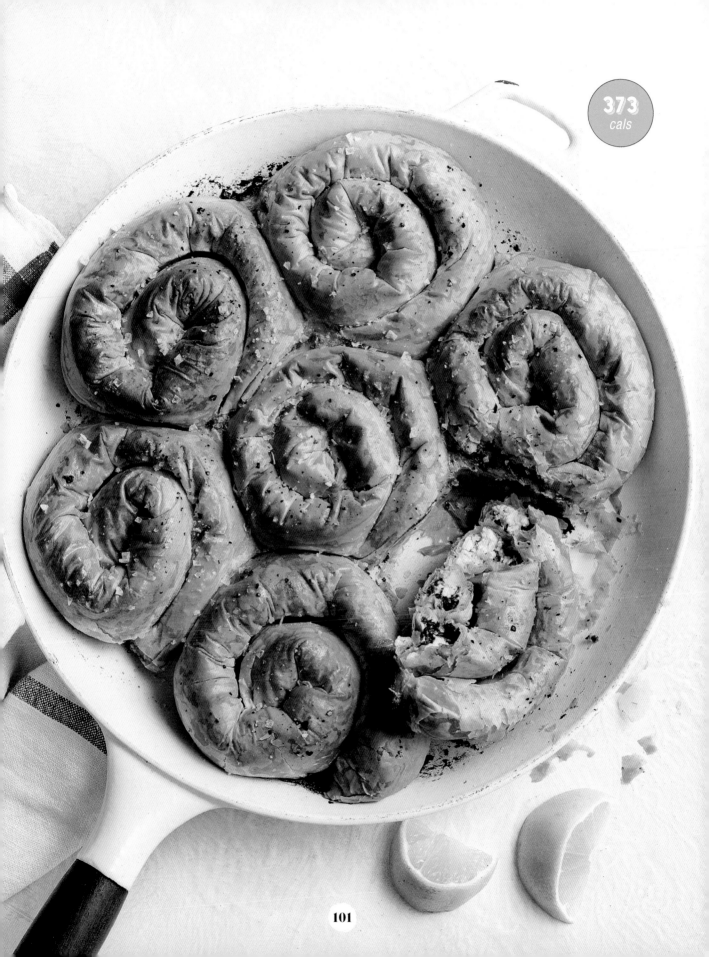

373
cals

# LEMONY TURMERIC & LENTIL SOUP

This healthy lentil vegetarian soup gets its lovely golden colour from turmeric, which contains curcumin, known for its anti-inflammatory properties.

**SERVES** 4 **PREP** 15 mins **COOK** 45 mins

2 tsp extra virgin olive oil
1 large red onion, finely chopped
3 celery sticks, finely chopped
2 garlic cloves, crushed
2 tsp finely grated lemon rind
1 tsp turmeric
½ tsp ground cinnamon
½ tsp dried chilli flakes
500ml (2 cups) vegetable stock
135g (¾ cup) French green lentils, rinsed, drained
2 vine-ripened tomatoes, chopped
150g green beans, trimmed, sliced
100g chopped kale
1 tbs fresh lemon juice
2 tbs chopped fresh coriander
Natural dairy-free yoghurt, to serve (optional)

1 Heat the olive oil in a large saucepan over medium heat. Add the onion and celery. Cook, stirring occasionally, for 5 minutes or until softened. Add the garlic, lemon rind, turmeric, cinnamon and chilli flakes. Cook, stirring, for 1 minute or until aromatic.

2 Add stock, lentils, tomato and 750ml (3 cups) water to the pan. Bring to the boil. Reduce the heat to low and partially cover. Simmer for 30 minutes, until lentils are tender.

3 Add the beans and kale to the soup. Stir to combine. Simmer for 3-4 minutes or until the beans are tender-crisp. Stir in the lemon juice and season with pepper. Stir in the coriander just before serving. Serve topped with a dollop of yoghurt, if you like.

## NUTRITION (PER SERVE)

| CALS | FAT | SAT FAT | PROTEIN | CARBS |
|------|-----|---------|---------|-------|
| 197  | 4g  | 1g      | 12g     | 24g   |

**COOK'S NOTE**

Did you know that many store-bought liquid and powdered stocks are vegetarian? Even if labelled chicken or beef, they may be just flavoured with vegetables and spices. Simply check the label before buying to be sure.

★★★★★ *I absolutely love this soup, deliciousness.* **TRIPPERMJ2**

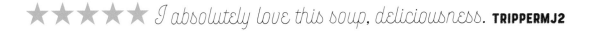

○ EASY   ○ FAMILY-FRIENDLY   ● **GLUTEN FREE**   ● **LOW CAL**   ○ QUICK   ● **VEGAN**

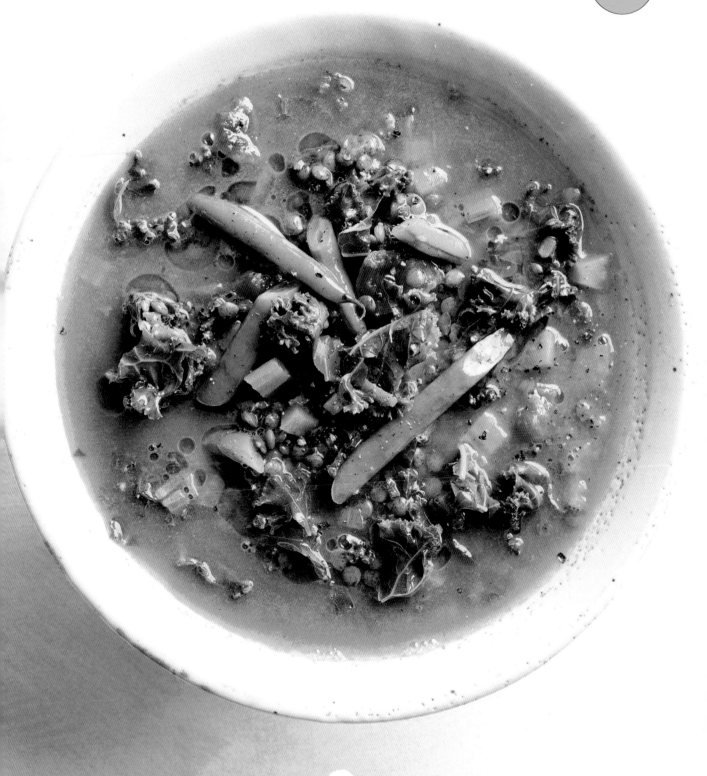

# HEALTHY POTATO-CRUST QUICHE

A potato hash brown base makes a great low-fat alternative to pastry in this healthy vegetarian quiche. The cheesy filling is a winner, too.

**SERVES** 6  **PREP** 20 mins  **COOK** 1 hour

750g coliban potatoes, peeled,
  coarsely grated
2 garlic cloves, crushed
1½ tbs extra virgin olive oil
1 large brown onion, chopped
1 large zucchini, coarsely grated
2 tsp finely grated lemon rind
120g trimmed kale, chopped
8 eggs
170g (⅔ cup) smooth ricotta
60g creamy feta, crumbled
2 tbs chopped fresh dill,
  plus extra, to serve
2 roma tomatoes, cut into
  thin wedges
Salad leaves and lemon wedges,
  to serve

1 Preheat oven to 200°C/180°C fan forced. Lightly spray a 24cm round tart tin or baking dish with olive oil. Use clean hands to squeeze out excess liquid from the potato. Combine the potato, half the garlic and 1 tbs oil in a large bowl. Press mixture firmly over base and side of prepared dish. Bake for 25 minutes or until golden.

2 Meanwhile, heat remaining oil in a large non-stick frying pan over medium heat. Add onion. Cook, stirring often, for 5 minutes or until softened. Use hands to squeeze out excess liquid from zucchini and add to the pan with the lemon rind and remaining garlic. Stir for 1 minute or until aromatic. Add kale. Cook, tossing occasionally, for 2 minutes or until just wilted.

3 Reduce oven to 180°C/160°C fan forced. Whisk the eggs and ricotta in a bowl. Stir in feta and dill. Season. Spoon kale mixture into the potato crust. Pour over the egg mixture. Top with tomato. Bake for 35 minutes or until filling is set and golden (cover edges with foil if browning too quickly). Set aside for 5 minutes to cool slightly. Top with extra dill and serve with salad leaves and lemon wedges.

**COOK'S NOTE**

Use this clever potato base as a gluten-free option for any of your favourite vegie quiche fillings.

## NUTRITION (PER SERVE)

| CALS | FAT | SAT FAT | PROTEIN | CARBS |
|------|-----|---------|---------|-------|
| 316 | 17g | 5.9g | 19.2g | 18.4g |

○ EASY  ● FAMILY-FRIENDLY  ● GLUTEN FREE  ● LOW CAL  ○ QUICK  ○ VEGAN

316
*cals*

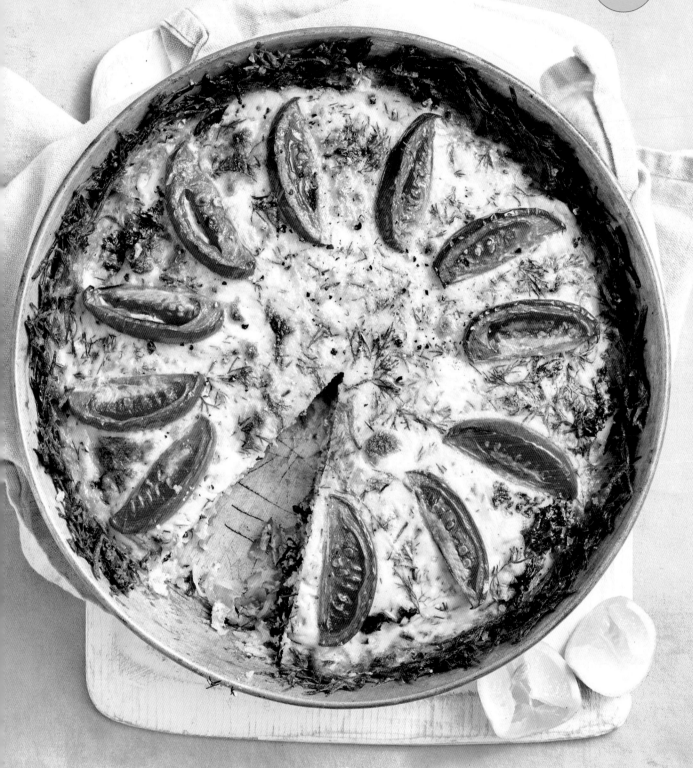

# SPRING RISONI-STUFFED
# CAPSICUMS

Looking for a healthy light meal or appetiser? These joyous stuffed capsicum halves are packed with loads of vegies and fresh herbs.

**SERVES** 8  **PREP** 15 mins  **COOK** 25 mins

4 small capsicums, halved lengthways, deseeded

60ml (¼ cup) olive oil, plus extra, to drizzle

2 bunches asparagus, cut into 2cm pieces

200g grape tomatoes, halved

1 garlic clove, thinly sliced

105g (½ cup) dried risoni pasta

1 small lemon, rind finely grated, juiced

⅔ cup fresh basil leaves

1 green shallot, thinly sliced

100g Greek-style feta, crumbled

85g (½ cup) Sicilian olives, pitted, coarsely chopped

Mixed salad leaves (otpional) and toasted pine nuts, to serve

1 Preheat oven to 220°C/200°C fan forced. Line 2 baking trays with baking paper. Place capsicum on 1 prepared tray, cut-side up, and brush with 1 tbs oil. Season. Toss the asparagus, tomato and garlic on the remaining prepared tray. Drizzle with 1 tbs oil. Season. Roast (with the capsicum on top shelf of oven) for 20-25 minutes or until capsicum is charred and all vegetables are tender.

2 Meanwhile, cook the pasta in a saucepan of salted boiling water for 8 minutes or until al dente. Drain. Refresh under cold running water. Combine the lemon rind, lemon juice and remaining oil in a large bowl. Finely chop 1 tbs basil and add to the bowl. Add the pasta, roasted vegetables, shallot, feta, olives and remaining basil. Season. Stir to combine.

3 Spoon risoni mixture among capsicums. Drizzle with extra oil and sprinkle with pine nuts, to serve.

**COOK'S NOTE**

Roast the capsicums and make the pasta salad, omitting basil, up to 1 day ahead. Store in separate airtight containers in the fridge. Stand salad at room temperature for 1 hour before tossing with the basil and stuffing the capsicums.

## NUTRITION (PER SERVE)

| CALS | FAT | SAT FAT | PROTEIN | CARBS |
|------|-----|---------|---------|-------|
| 256.5 | 17.3g | 3.5g | 7.7g | 15.3g |

● EASY  ○ FAMILY-FRIENDLY  ○ GLUTEN FREE  ● LOW CAL  ○ QUICK  ○ VEGAN

257
cals

★★★★★
I served these as a starter at a barbecue and they were a hit!
It didn't matter if the people were vegetarian or not, these stuffed
beauties were loved by all. SHAWNSALAD

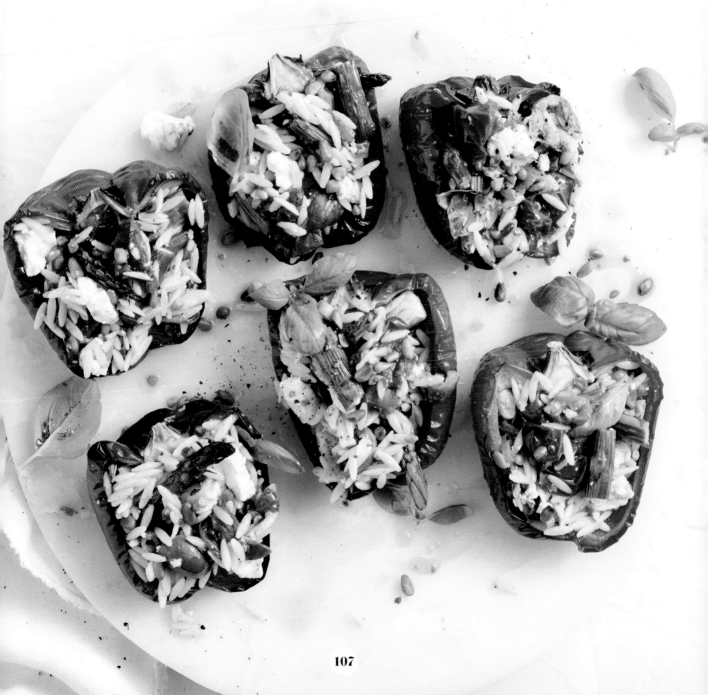

# 'BACON' & SWEET POTATO
# SPAGHETTI

We've given this vegan salad with sweet potato spaghetti a delicious smoky bacon flavour by tossing in cubes of haloumi coated in smoked paprika.

**SERVES** 4  **PREP** 15 mins  **COOK** 15 mins

250g tomato medley mix, halved
500g sweet potato noodles
   (see note)
1 tsp smoked paprika
1 tsp nutritional yeast
180g salt-reduced haloumi,
   cut into 1.5cm pieces
1 tsp extra virgin olive oil
2 garlic cloves, thinly sliced
2 tsp finely grated lemon rind
2 bunches broccolini, cut into
   4cm lengths
½ cup fresh small basil leaves
Lemon wedges, to serve

1 Preheat the oven to 170°C/150°C fan forced. Grease a large baking tray and line with baking paper. Spread tomato over the prepared tray and lightly spray with olive oil. Bake for 12 minutes or until just wrinkled.

2 Meanwhile, place noodles in a large microwave-safe bowl. Microwave, covered, for 6 minutes or until tender. Drain.

3 Combine paprika and yeast in a small bowl. Sprinkle evenly over the haloumi and set aside.

4 Heat the oil in a large frying pan over medium heat. Add garlic and lemon rind and cook, stirring, for 30 seconds or until aromatic. Add broccolini and 2 tbs water. Cook, stirring, for 3 minutes or until broccolini is just tender.

5 Add noodles and tomato to the frying pan and gently toss to combine. Season. Cover to keep warm.

6 Heat a separate frying pan over high heat and spray lightly with olive oil. Cook haloumi for 30 seconds each side or until golden. Divide noodle mixture among serving bowls and top with smoky haloumi. Sprinkle with basil. Serve with lemon wedges for squeezing over.

## COOK'S NOTE

Also called sweet potato spaghetti, look for them in the fresh produce section of supermarkets, or use a spiraliser to cut noodles from 500g peeled sweet potato.

## NUTRITION (PER SERVE)

| CALS | FAT | SAT FAT | PROTEIN | CARBS |
|------|-----|---------|---------|-------|
| 309 | 14g | 8g | 15g | 24g |

● EASY  ○ FAMILY-FRIENDLY  ● GLUTEN FREE  ● LOW CAL  ● QUICK  ○ VEGAN

309
*cals*

★★★★★
*I made this for lunch today – absolutely sensational.*
*A bit light for dinner, perhaps, but as it stands, it is a beautiful dish!*

**COOKINGMAMA1902**

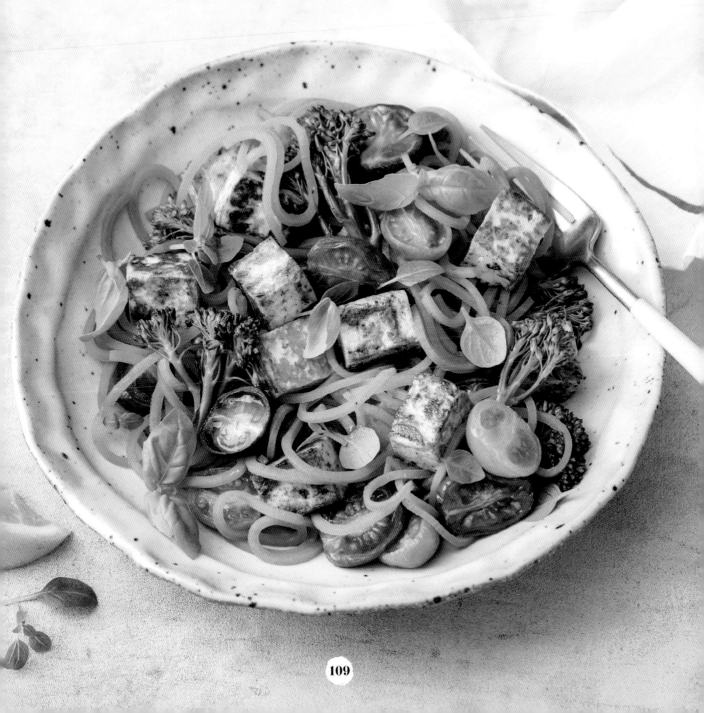

# SPICY MEXICAN POLENTA MUFFINS

These low-cal gluten-free muffins pack a little Mexican heat. We've also given them a vitamin boost with a mashed avo and crunchy salsa topping.

**MAKES** 9 **PREP** 20 mins **COOK** 25 mins

150g (1 cup) gluten-free
   self-raising flour
2 tsp gluten-free baking powder
170g (1 cup) fine polenta
1 long fresh red chilli, deseeded,
   finely chopped
4 green shallots, finely chopped
285g (1½ cups) fresh corn kernels
200g jar roasted red capsicum
   (not in oil), coarsely chopped
2 eggs
2 tbs extra virgin olive oil
125ml (½ cup) unsweetened
   almond milk
70g feta, crumbled
Mashed avocado and coriander
   leaves (optional), to serve

**1** Preheat oven to 190°C/170°C fan forced. Line nine 185ml (¾ cup) muffin pans with paper cases. Sift the flour and baking powder into a large bowl. Stir in polenta, chilli, shallot, 185g (1 cup) corn, and three-quarters of the capsicum. Combine the remaining corn and capsicum in a bowl and set aside.

**2** Whisk the eggs, oil and milk in a jug. Add to the polenta mixture and stir until just combined. Stir through feta.

**3** Divide mixture among prepared muffin pans. Bake for 20-25 minutes or until muffins are golden and a skewer inserted into the centres comes out clean. Serve warm or at room temperature topped with avocado, the corn and capsicum salsa and sprinkled with coriander, if desired.

**COOK'S NOTE**

Corn and polenta (also made from corn) is rich in the carotenoid lutein, known to assist eye health and prevent macular degeneration.

## NUTRITION (PER SERVE)

| CALS | FAT | SAT FAT | PROTEIN | CARBS |
|------|-----|---------|---------|-------|
| 229 | 7.9g | 2.2g | 6.1g | 32.2g |

★★★★★ *These muffins were a little spicy, but not overwhelming. We really enjoyed adding the avocado and salsa.* **SHAWNSALAD**

● EASY   ○ FAMILY-FRIENDLY   ● GLUTEN FREE   ● LOW CAL   ○ QUICK   ○ VEGAN

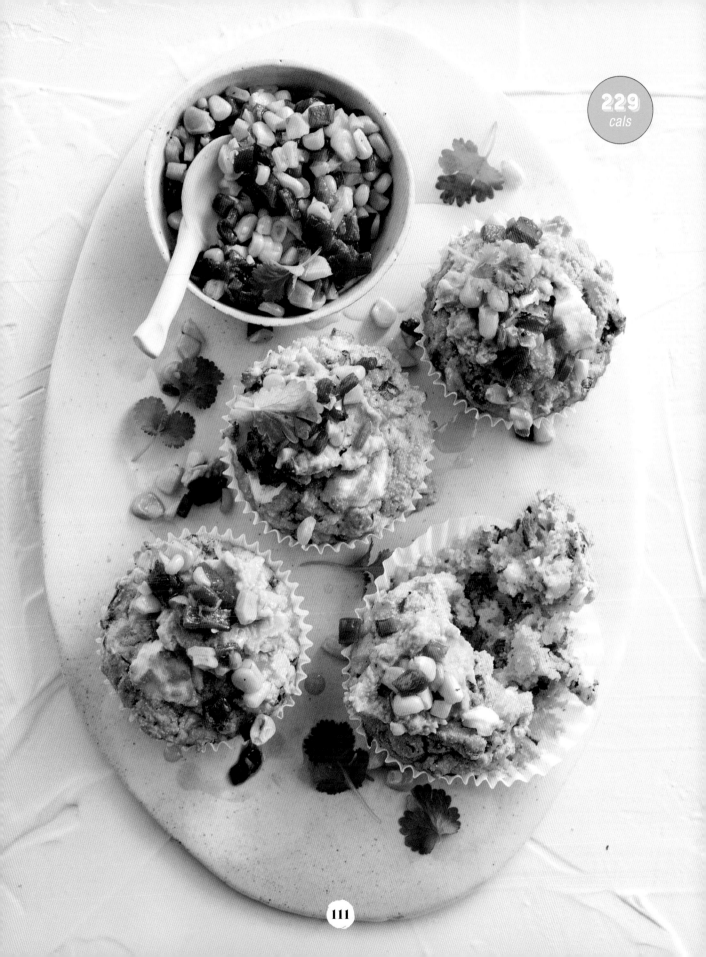

229
cals

# EGGPLANT, FETA & QUINOA SALAD

High in iron and protein, quinoa is a great alternative to meat. Tossed with roasted vegies in this aromatic warm salad, it's super easy to eat healthy.

**SERVES** 4  **PREP** 20 mins  **COOK** 20 mins

1 eggplant, cut into 2cm pieces
2 red onions, halved, cut into thin wedges
1 large zucchini, cut into 2cm pieces
250g small cherry tomatoes
1 tsp olive oil
1 garlic clove, crushed
1 tsp ground cumin
200g (1 cup) tricolour quinoa
500ml (2 cups) water
400g can no-added-salt chickpeas, rinsed, drained
½ cup fresh basil leaves, torn
50g low-fat feta, crumbled
2 tsp extra virgin olive oil
Balsamic vinegar, to drizzle
Fresh basil leaves, extra, to serve

1 Preheat oven to 200°C/180°C fan forced. Line a large baking tray with baking paper. Place the eggplant, onion and zucchini on the prepared tray. Spray with oil and season with pepper. Roast for 10 minutes. Add the tomatoes and roast for 10 minutes or until all vegetables are golden and tender.

2 Meanwhile, heat the olive oil in a saucepan over medium heat. Stir in the garlic and cumin for 30 seconds or until aromatic. Add the quinoa and water. Bring to the boil. Reduce heat to low. Cover and simmer for 12 minutes or until the quinoa is tender and the water has absorbed. Set aside to cool slightly.

3 Place the quinoa, roasted vegetables, chickpeas, basil and feta in a large bowl. Toss gently to combine. Divide among serving bowls and drizzle with oil and vinegar. Sprinkle with basil, to serve.

**COOK'S NOTE**

Why quinoa? It contains as much iron as meat, is a good source of protein and fibre, has the five B vitamins (B1, B2, B3, B6 and folate), as well as vitamin E.

## NUTRITION (PER SERVE)

| CALS | FAT | SAT FAT | PROTEIN | CARBS |
|------|-----|---------|---------|-------|
| 370  | 11g | 2g      | 18g     | 50g   |

● EASY   ○ FAMILY-FRIENDLY   ● GLUTEN FREE   ● LOW CAL   ○ QUICK   ○ VEGAN

370 cals

★ ★ ★ ★ ★
*Loved this! Simple to make, super tasty and very filling!
This one's going in the repertoire :).* **CLBARBER**

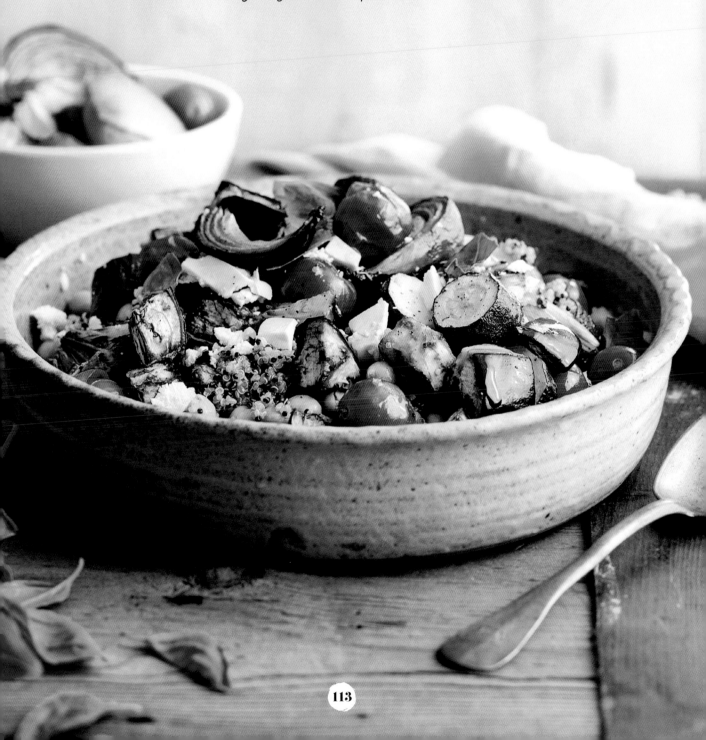

113

# WARMING ROASTED PUMPKIN SOUP

Packed with health-giving spices, such as ginger and turmeric, you'll feel on top of the world after a ladle of this easy and delicious soup.

**SERVES** 4  **PREP** 25 mins  **COOK** 1 hour 25 mins

1.6kg butternut pumpkin or
   kent pumpkin
60ml (¼ cup) olive oil
1 large brown onion, finely chopped
2 garlic cloves, finely chopped
1L (4 cups) gluten-free chicken stock
1 tbs finely grated fresh ginger
1 tbs finely grated fresh turmeric
   (see note)
Natural yoghurt and mixed baby
   herbs (such as coriander, purple
   radish sprouts), to serve

1 Preheat oven to 200°C/180°C fan forced. Line 2 baking trays with baking paper. Coarsely chop the pumpkin, discarding the seeds. Spread over the prepared trays. Drizzle with 2 tbs oil. Bake for 1 hour 10 minutes or until pumpkin is soft and lightly coloured.

2 Meanwhile, heat the remaining oil in a large, heavy-based saucepan over medium heat. Add the onion. Cook, stirring, for 3-5 minutes or until slightly softened. Add the garlic and cook, stirring, for 1 minute or until aromatic.

3 Remove skin from the cooked pumpkin and add to the pan with any juices from the tray. Stir in the stock. Bring to a simmer over medium-low heat. Simmer for 15 minutes. Stir in the ginger and turmeric. Remove from the heat. Use a stick blender to puree mixture until smooth, thinning with a little water, if you prefer. Ladle soup among serving bowls. Serve topped with a dollop of yoghurt and the baby herbs.

## COOK'S NOTE

Fresh turmeric is a rich source of antioxidants. Pick it up at good greengrocers or substitute with 1 tsp ground turmeric. Garnishing the soup with yoghurt instead of cream lowers the calories and adds a probiotic boost.

## NUTRITION (PER SERVE)

| CALS | FAT | SAT FAT | PROTEIN | CARBS |
|------|-----|---------|---------|-------|
| 373 | 19g | 9g | 16g | 31g |

● EASY  ● FAMILY-FRIENDLY  ● GLUTEN FREE  ● LOW CAL  ○ QUICK  ○ VEGAN

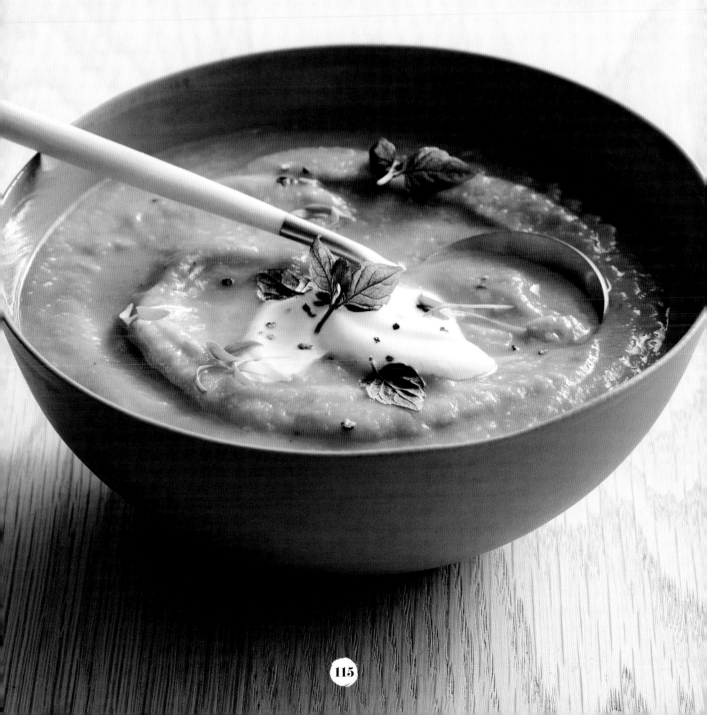

373
cals

★ ★ ★ ★ ★

*Lovely soup. Just a little interesting twist on the usual pumpkin soup. This will be my go-to soup recipe from now on.* **ROSEBUD23**

# JAPANESE STUFFED SWEET POTATOES

Add some miso to your roasted sweet potatoes for an easy, low-cal and plant-based dinner that's as colourful as it is thoroughly delicious.

**SERVES** 4  **PREP** 15 mins  **COOK** 50 mins

4 small (about 200g each) scrubbed
  sweet potatoes (see note)
1½ tbs mirin
1 tbs miso paste
2 tsp salt-reduced, gluten-free
  soy sauce
1 tsp sesame oil
250g firm tofu, cut into 1cm cubes
145g (1 cup) podded
  frozen edamame
¼ small red cabbage, shredded
4 green shallots, thinly sliced
2 tsp finely grated fresh ginger
2 tsp toasted sesame seeds

**1** Preheat the oven to 200°C/180°C fan forced. Use a fork or skewer to prick sweet potatoes all over. Place on a baking tray and roast, turning once, for 50 minutes or until tender when pierced.

**2** Meanwhile, combine the mirin, miso, soy sauce and oil in a jug. Lightly spray a non-stick wok with olive oil and heat over high heat. Cook tofu, in 2 batches, stirring, for 2-3 minutes or until golden. Transfer to a plate. Reduce heat to medium-high and spray wok with a little more oil. Add edamame, cabbage, shallot and ginger. Cook, stirring, for 2 minutes or until just tender. Return tofu to the wok with half the miso mixture and stir for 1 minute or until heated through.

**3** Cut a long slit along each potato. Use a fork to lightly mash flesh. Spoon filling into each potato. Top with remaining miso mixture and sesame seeds, to serve.

## COOK'S NOTE

Using the sweet potatoes, skin and all, means nothing gets thrown away and your body gets to enjoy extra nutrients. Just be sure to wash them well before roasting.

## NUTRITION (PER SERVE)

| CALS | FAT | SAT FAT | PROTEIN | CARBS |
|------|-----|---------|---------|-------|
| 345 | 10.3g | 1.4g | 18g | 39.4g |

○ EASY  ● FAMILY-FRIENDLY  ● GLUTEN FREE  ● LOW CAL  ○ QUICK  ● VEGAN

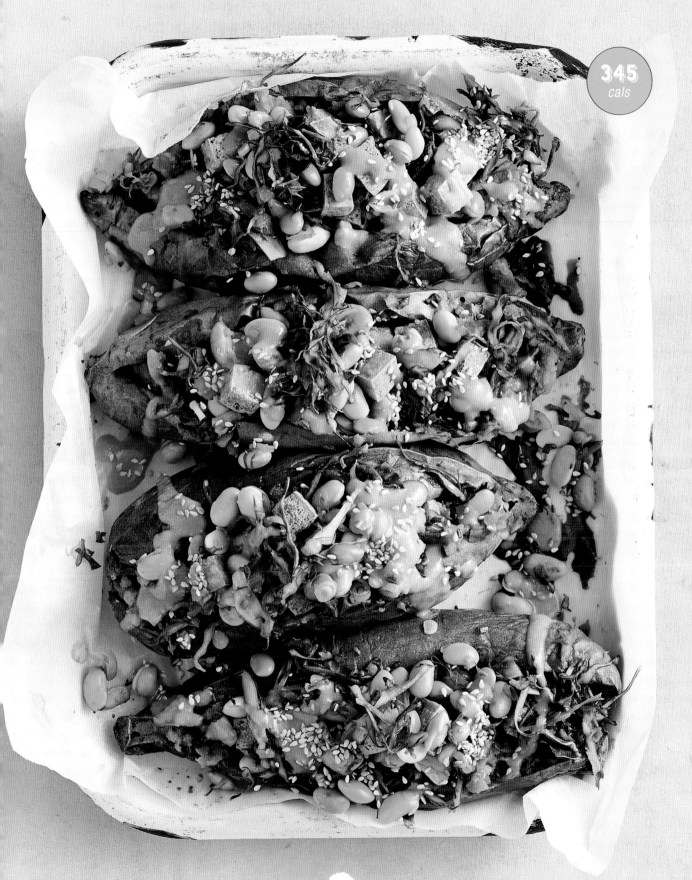

345
cals

# RED CABBAGE WITH PUMPKIN FALAFEL

Try these flavour-packed pumpkin falafels nestled in a glorious red cabbage salad and drizzled in a creamy feta dressing. Yum!

**SERVES** 4  **PREP** 20 mins (+ cooling & chilling)  **COOK** 55 mins

300g kent pumpkin, peeled, deseeded, cut into 2cm pieces
1 bunch baby carrots, trimmed, peeled
½ red onion, cut into wedges
1 tbs extra virgin olive oil
400g can chickpeas, rinsed, drained
2 garlic cloves, chopped
½ cup fresh coriander leaves
1 lemon, rind finely grated, juiced
1-2 tsp harissa paste, to taste
60g (1 cup) fresh gluten-free breadcrumbs
68g (¼ cup) Persian-style feta dip
1 tbs warm water
250g red cabbage, finely shredded
50g finely shredded kale
150g cooked beetroot, coarsely chopped

1. Preheat oven to 180°C/160°C fan forced. Line a large baking tray with baking paper. Arrange the pumpkin, carrot and onion on the prepared tray. Drizzle over oil. Season. Roast for 35 minutes or until tender. Cool.

2. Place chickpeas, garlic, coriander, lemon rind, harissa, pumpkin and onion in a food processor. Pulse until just combined. Season. Add the breadcrumbs and pulse to combine. Roll 2 tbs mixture at a time to make balls. Flatten slightly. Place on a plate. Place in the fridge for 10 minutes to firm up a little.

3. Spray a frying pan with oil. Cook falafel, in 3 batches, for 3 minutes each side or until golden and heated through.

4. Combine the dip, lemon juice and water in a jug. Place cabbage and kale in a bowl. Toss with half the dressing. Season. Transfer to a serving plate. Top with the carrots, beetroot, falafel, remaining dressing and pepitas, to serve.

**COOK'S NOTE**

Red cabbage is a good source of fibre and potassium, and has a higher level of vitamin C than the white and green varieties.

**NUTRITION** (PER SERVE)

| CALS | FAT | SAT FAT | PROTEIN | CARBS |
|------|-----|---------|---------|-------|
| 360 | 5g | 19g | 13g | 27g |

○ EASY  ○ FAMILY-FRIENDLY  ● GLUTEN FREE  ● LOW CAL  ○ QUICK  ○ VEGAN

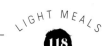

360 cals

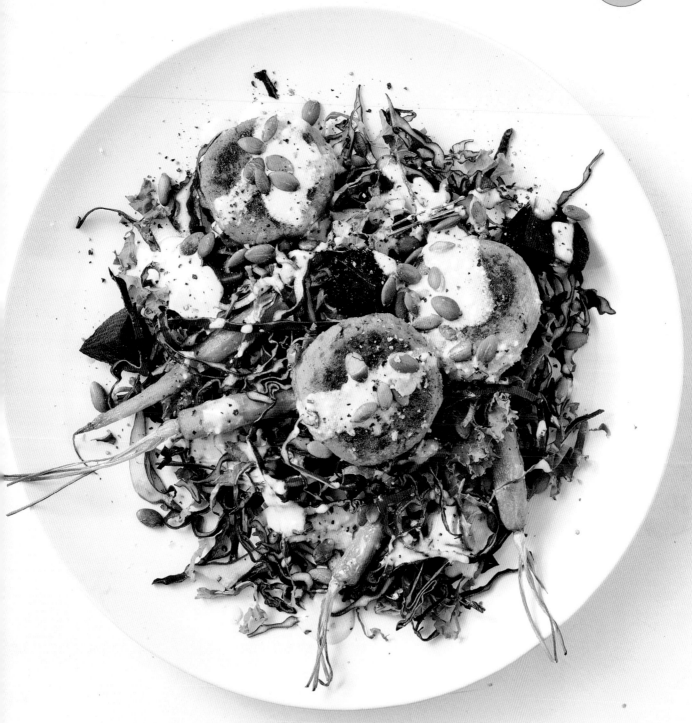

# LOADED CHICKPEA PANCAKES

Made with chickpea flour, these pancakes are gluten free and full of fibre. Load them up with hummus and whatever vegies you have on hand.

**SERVES** 4  **PREP** 15 mins (+30 mins standing)  **COOK** 25 mins

120g chickpea (besan) flour
250ml (1 cup) warm water
2 zucchini, halved lengthways, cut into 5mm-thick slices
1 large red capsicum, deseeded, thickly sliced
250g button mushrooms, halved
200g peeled pumpkin, thinly sliced
1 tbs extra virgin olive oil
4 eggs
80g (⅓ cup) hummus
80g baby spinach
Sriracha chilli sauce, to serve
Fresh micro herbs or baby rocket, to serve (optional)

1 Place the flour and a large pinch of salt in a bowl. Gradually whisk in the warm water until smooth. Set aside for 30 minutes to thicken slightly. Transfer to a jug.

2 Preheat a barbecue grill or chargrill pan on medium-high. Lightly spray zucchini, capsicum, mushroom and pumpkin with olive oil. Grill capsicum, mushroom and pumpkin for 2-3 minutes each side and zucchini for 1-2 minutes each side or until tender and lightly charred.

3 Heat 1 tsp oil in a non-stick frying pan over high heat. Add one-quarter of the pancake mixture, swirling to coat base. Cook for 1-2 minutes or until bubbles appear. Turn over and cook for 1-2 minutes or until golden. Transfer to a plate. Repeat with remaining oil and pancake mixture to make 4 pancakes.

4 Meanwhile, lightly spray a large non-stick frying pan with olive oil. Heat over medium-high heat. Fry eggs for 3-4 minutes or until cooked to your liking.

5 Place pancakes on serving plates. Spread with 1 tbs hummus. Top with the veg, an egg and spinach. Drizzle over sriracha. Sprinkle with herbs or rocket, if using. Serve.

**COOK'S NOTE**

For a vegan version, drop the eggs and add some sliced avocado with a squeeze of lemon juice.

## NUTRITION (PER SERVE)

| CALS | FAT | SAT FAT | PROTEIN | CARBS |
|------|-----|---------|---------|-------|
| 378 | 20.5g | 3.4g | 19g | 22.6g |

○ EASY  ○ FAMILY-FRIENDLY  ● GLUTEN FREE  ● LOW CAL  ○ QUICK  ○ VEGAN

378 cals

★ ★ ★ ★ ★

*This is a nice change from regular pancakes, and the fact they are better for you is a bonus!* **SHAWNSALAD**

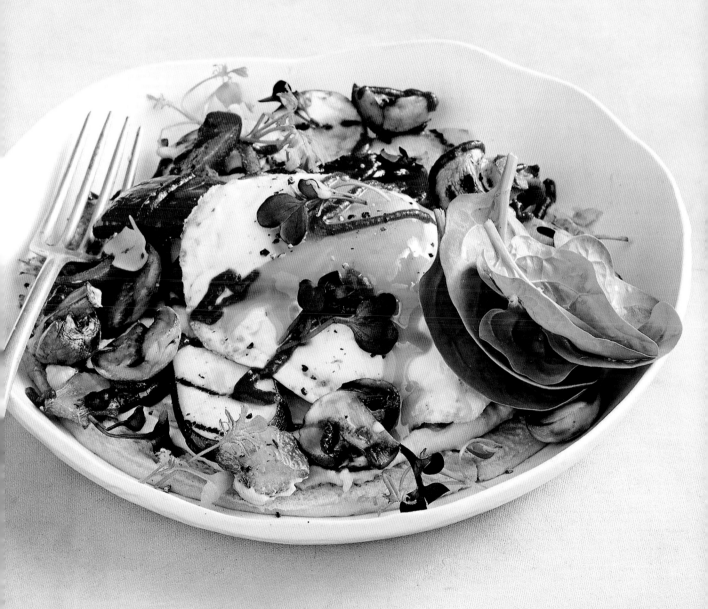

# MAIN MEALS

LOAD UP ON PROTEIN AND VEG WITH HEARTIER DISHES.
THEY'RE ALL UNDER 600 CALORIES PER SERVE!

# MUSHROOM & LENTIL LASAGNE

Mushrooms lend their meaty flavour and texture to this veg-packed, protein-rich lasagne. Trust us, meat eaters will love this dish, too!

**SERVES** 6  **PREP** 30 mins  **COOK** 1 hour 15 mins

2 tbs olive oil
1 brown onion, finely chopped
1 carrot, finely chopped
2 small celery sticks,
  finely chopped
300g button mushrooms, sliced
2 garlic cloves, crushed
2 tbs tomato paste
2 x 400g cans brown lentils,
  rinsed, drained
400g can diced tomatoes
250ml (1 cup) vegetable stock
1 tsp dried Italian herbs
200g flat mushrooms, thinly sliced
6-8 fresh lasagne sheets
**WHITE SAUCE**
30g butter
1½ tbs plain flour
375ml (1½ cups) milk
155g (1½ cups) grated cheddar

**1** Preheat oven to 200°C/180°C fan forced. Grease a 2L (8 cup) baking dish. Heat the oil in a large deep frying pan over medium heat. Add the onion, carrot and celery. Cook, stirring occasionally, for 10 minutes or until golden. Add button mushrooms and cook, stirring, for 3-4 minutes or until softened. Add garlic and cook, stirring, for 30 seconds or until aromatic. Stir in tomato paste, lentils, tomato, stock and herbs. Bring to a simmer. Reduce heat to low. Simmer for 5 minutes or until thickened. Season. Transfer to a bowl.

**2** Heat a clean large frying pan over medium-high heat. Spray flat mushroom with olive oil. Cook, in batches, for 2 minutes each side or until browned. Transfer to a plate. Line base of the prepared dish with pasta, cutting sheets to fit, as needed. Spread one-third of the lentil mixture over the pasta. Top with another layer of pasta and half the remaining lentil mixture. Repeat with pasta and remaining lentil mixture. Top with a final layer of pasta.

**3** For the white sauce, melt butter in a saucepan over medium heat. Add the flour and cook, stirring, for 2 minutes. Gradually whisk in the milk until smooth. Bring to the boil and cook, stirring occasionally, for 2 minutes until thickened. Add 100g (1 cup) cheese and cook, stirring until melted and smooth. Season.

**4** Spread the white sauce over the top layer of pasta and sprinkle with remaining cheese. Arrange the flat mushroom over the top. Bake for 40 minutes or until golden. Set aside for 10 minutes to cool slightly, before serving.

## NUTRITION (PER SERVE)

| CALS | FAT | SAT FAT | PROTEIN | CARBS |
|------|-----|---------|---------|-------|
| 484 | 21.8g | 9.7g | 22g | 46.4g |

○ EASY  ● FAMILY-FRIENDLY  ○ GLUTEN FREE  ● LOW CAL  ○ QUICK  ○ VEGAN

484
*cals*

★ ★ ★ ★ ★

*This was delicious! The flavours were divine and the white sauce topping was sooo creamy. Will make it again, for sure.* **SHAWNTHEPRAWN**

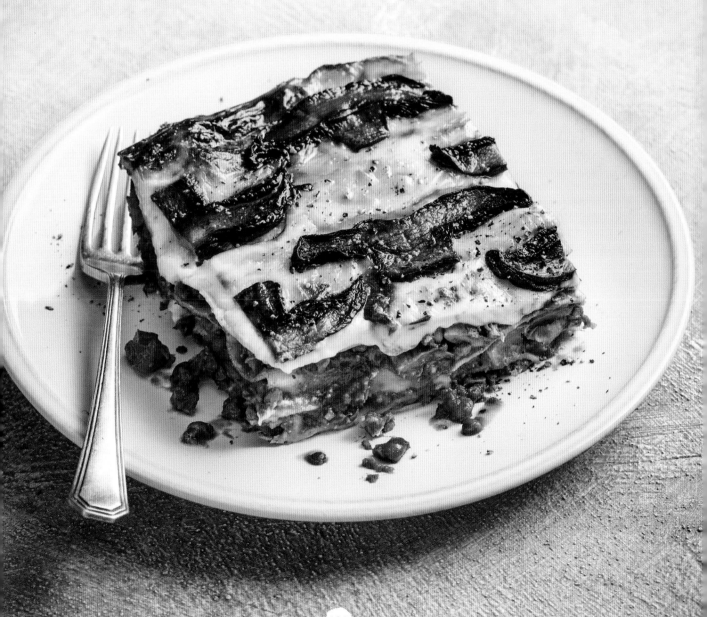

# QUICK VEGETARIAN
# MINESTRONE

We think minestrone is the perfect mid-week soup – it uses pantry staples, it's fast and it's healthy. Here's our super-speedy take on it.

**SERVES** 4 **PREP** 15 mins **COOK** 35 mins

2 tbs olive oil, plus extra, to drizzle
1 leek, halved, thinly sliced
3 garlic cloves, 2 crushed, 1 halved
1 rosemary sprig
500g root vegetables, chopped
   (see note)
1 tbs tomato paste
1L (4 cups) vegetable stock
400g can diced tomatoes
400g can borlotti beans, rinsed,
   drained
80g dried thin spaghetti, broken
60g pkt baby kale
4 slices sourdough bread

1 Heat the oil in a large saucepan over medium heat. Add the leek, crushed garlic and rosemary sprig. Cook, stirring, for 3 minutes or until aromatic. Add the root vegies and cook, stirring, for 3 minutes or until slightly softened. Add the tomato paste. Cook, stirring, for 1 minute.

2 Add the stock and tomato. Cover. Bring to the boil. Simmer for 15 minutes or until vegies are softened. Add beans and pasta. Cook, stirring occasionally, for 8 minutes or until pasta is al dente. Add kale. Cook, stirring, until wilted.

3 Toast bread. Rub with garlic. Drizzle with olive oil and season. Serve garlic toast with the soup.

**COOK'S NOTE**

Use a mixture of vegies such as sweet potato, swede, turnip and carrot. You could also add pumpkin or potato, if you desire.

## NUTRITION (PER SERVE)

| CALS | FAT | SAT FAT | PROTEIN | CARBS |
|------|-----|---------|---------|-------|
| 475 | 16.7g | 2.8g | 15.4g | 62.5g |

★★★★★ *This was surprisingly easy to make, and filled with wonderful flavours. So warming!* **MURRAYMINT**

● EASY  ● FAMILY-FRIENDLY  ○ GLUTEN FREE  ● LOW CAL  ○ QUICK  ● VEGAN

475
cals

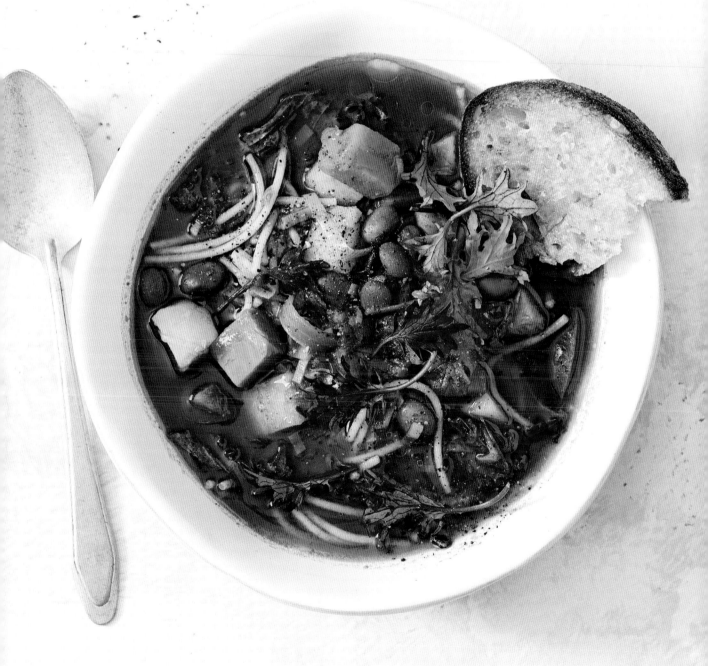

# VEGAN CHICKPEA SATAY CURRY

Ready in 30 minutes, this creamy chickpea curry is also loaded with pumpkin and cooked in a delicious peanut butter and coconut milk sauce.

**SERVES** 4  **PREP** 15 mins  **COOK** 15 mins

1 tbs peanut oil
1 brown onion, cut into thin wedges
2 garlic cloves, crushed
1 tsp crushed red chilli
   (or sambal oelek)
90g (⅓ cup) smooth peanut butter
160ml (⅔ cup) coconut milk
2 tbs light gluten-free soy sauce
700g pumpkin, peeled, deseeded,
   cut into 2cm pieces
160ml (⅔ cup) water
200g green beans, trimmed, halved
400g can chickpeas, drained, rinsed
1 tbs fresh lime juice
¼ cup fresh coriander leaves
Steamed brown rice, to serve

1 Heat the oil in a large, deep frying pan or wok over medium heat. Add the onion and cook, stirring occasionally, for 5 minutes or until softened and lightly golden. Add the garlic and chilli. Cook, stirring, for 30 seconds or until aromatic.

2 Reduce heat to low. Add the peanut butter, coconut milk and soy sauce, stirring to combine. Add the pumpkin and water. Cover and bring to a simmer. Cook, stirring occasionally, for 6 minutes or until pumpkin is just tender.

3 Add the beans and chickpeas to the pan. Cook for 2 minutes or until beans are tender-crisp. Stir in the lime juice and top with coriander. Serve with brown rice.

**COOK'S NOTE**

Use peanut butter with no added sugar or salt, if you like.

## NUTRITION (PER SERVE)

| CALS | FAT | SAT FAT | PROTEIN | CARBS |
|------|-----|---------|---------|-------|
| 527 | 25.5g | 9g | 17g | 51.5g |

● EASY  ● FAMILY-FRIENDLY  ● GLUTEN FREE  ● LOW CAL  ● QUICK  ● VEGAN

527
*cals*

★ ★ ★ ★ ★
*I loved making this, it was so quick and easy and tasted delicious.* **MHARTIG**

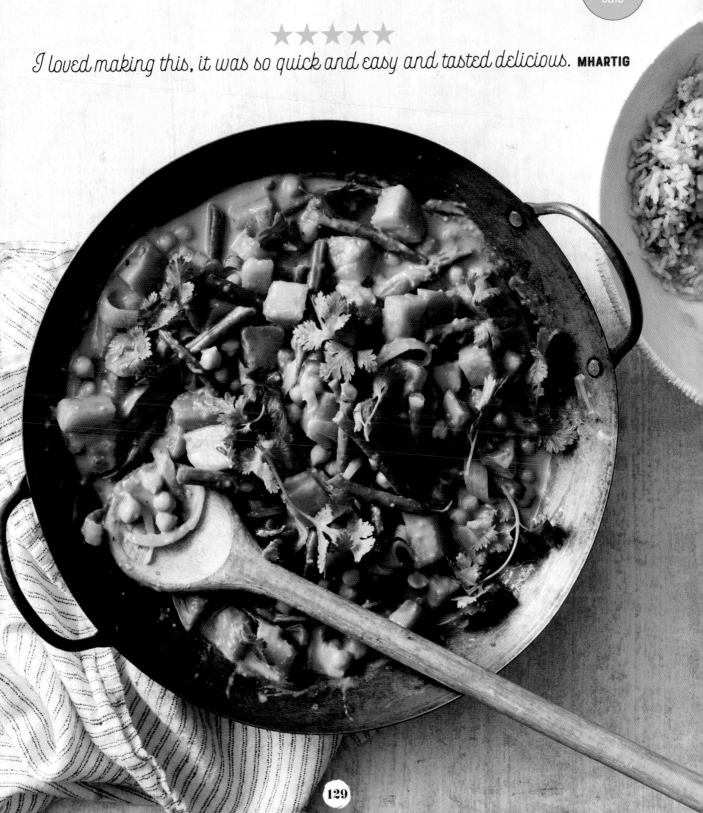

# MEXICAN TACO

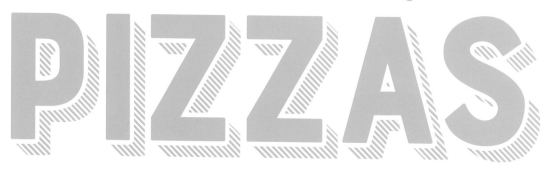

# PIZZAS

Taco meets pizza in this quick and easy vegetarian family dinner fix.
Go ahead and add as much chilli and hot sauce as your palate can handle!

**SERVES** 4  **PREP** 5 mins  **COOK** 15 mins

2 x 440g (2-pack) pizza bases
300g jar medium chunky salsa
425g can pinto beans, rinsed, drained
100g (1 cup) grated mozzarella or
    pizza cheese
200g cherry tomatoes, halved
1 small red onion, sliced
Sour cream, hot sauce, sliced
    avocado, fresh coriander sprigs,
    sliced fresh chilli and lime wedges,
    to serve

**1** Preheat the oven to 220°C/200°C fan forced. Place the pizza bases on 2 large baking trays. Spread bases with the salsa. Place the beans in a bowl, lightly mash, then spread over the top of the salsa.

**2** Sprinkle a quarter of the cheese over each pizza. Top with the tomato and onion. Sprinkle with the remaining cheese. Bake pizzas for 10-15 minutes or until the cheese is melted and golden.

**3** Top each pizza with sour cream, hot sauce, avocado, coriander sprigs and chilli. Serve with lime wedges for squeezing over.

### COOK'S NOTE

You can use other canned beans, such as cannellini, kidney or borlotti beans, instead of the pinto beans, if you prefer.

## NUTRITION (PER SERVE)

| CALS | FAT | SAT FAT | PROTEIN | CARBS |
|------|-----|---------|---------|-------|
| 585 | 23.4g | 4.6g | 8g | 69g |

★★★★★ *What a fun family recipe! My kids even volunteered to help me in the kitchen.* **CHARLIEDINNER**

● EASY  ● FAMILY-FRIENDLY  ○ GLUTEN FREE  ● LOW CAL  ● QUICK  ○ VEGAN

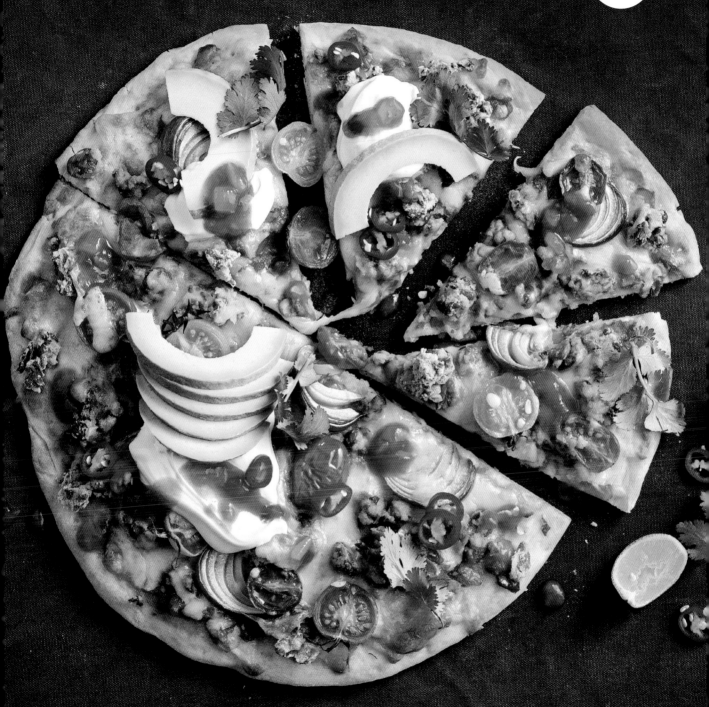

# CHEESY-STUFFED CAULIFLOWER

For a vegetarian main that is sure to impress, you can't beat this whole roasted cauliflower stuffed with feta and covered in a zucchini lattice.

**SERVES** 6  **PREP** 20 mins (+ cooling)  **COOK** 1 hour 10 mins

1 (about 1.2 kg) whole cauliflower, leaves removed
1 tbs olive oil
4 green shallots, thinly sliced
2 garlic cloves, crushed
60g pkt baby spinach, chopped
2 large zucchini
100g creamy feta, crumbled
2 tsp finely grated lemon rind
1 tsp finely chopped fresh thyme leaves
1 egg, lightly beaten
25g (½ cup) panko breadcrumbs
25g (⅓ cup) finely grated parmesan
Sweet paprika, to sprinkle

1. Preheat oven to 190°C/170°C fan forced. Line 2 baking trays with baking paper. Trim the base of the cauliflower so it sits flat. Place, cut-side up, in a microwave-safe bowl. Drizzle over 2 tbs water and microwave for 8 minutes or until just tender. Uncover and set aside to cool.

2. Heat the oil in a frying pan over medium heat. Add the shallot and cook, stirring occasionally, for 2 minutes or until softened. Add the garlic and cook, stirring, for 1 minute or until aromatic. Add the spinach and cook, stirring, for 1 minute or until wilted. Transfer to a bowl and set aside to cool.

3. Meanwhile, use a sharp knife or mandolin to cut the zucchini lengthways into 4mm-thick slices. Arrange slices in a lattice pattern on 1 prepared tray and spray with oil. Bake for 10 minutes or until softened slightly. Set aside to cool.

4. Add the feta, lemon rind, thyme and egg to the spinach mixture. Season with pepper and stir to combine. Fold in the breadcrumbs.

5. Turn the cauliflower upside down and poke the spinach mixture into the spaces between the florets. Use a chopstick or skewer to push in the mixture where your fingers can't reach. Place the cauliflower, right-side up, on the remaining prepared tray and sprinkle with 1 tbs parmesan.

6. Carefully place the zucchini lattice on top of the cauliflower to cover. Spray with oil. Cover loosely with foil and bake for 40 minutes. Uncover, sprinkle with remaining parmesan and a little paprika. Cook, uncovered, for 15 minutes or until golden and tender. Cut into wedges to serve.

## NUTRITION (PER SERVE)

| CALS | FAT | SAT FAT | PROTEIN | CARBS |
|------|-----|---------|---------|-------|
| 186 | 9.8g | 4g | 11.1g | 11.5g |

○ EASY  ○ FAMILY-FRIENDLY  ○ GLUTEN FREE  ● LOW CAL  ○ QUICK  ○ VEGAN

★ ★ ★ ★ ★

*This looked good in the photo, and tasted really good, too. My carnivore husband loved it! It was a bit tricky stuffing the filling into the cauliflower; fingers are the go.* **PJ**

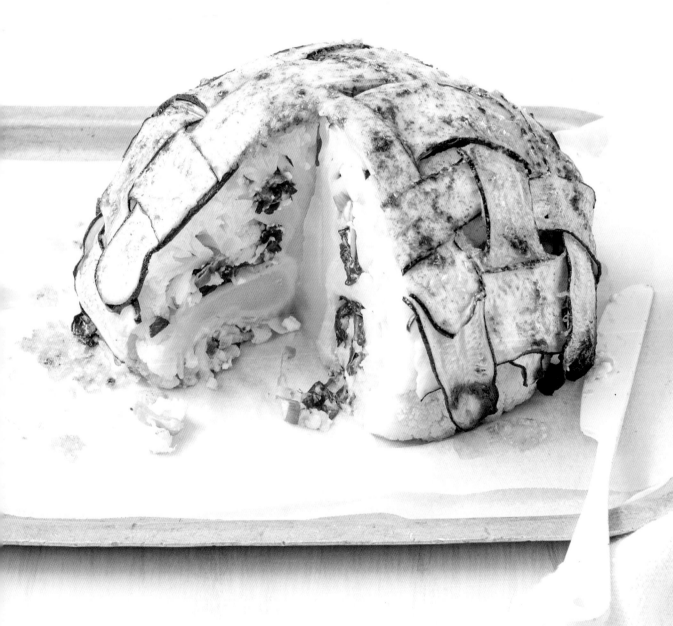

# ONE-PAN VEGETABLE
# BIRYANI

Keep midweek dinners fuss-free. There's no need for a grocery run when you can whip up this hearty vego dinner with what's in the fridge!

**SERVES** 6  **PREP** 20 mins (+ standing)  **COOK** 25 mins

20g butter
2 tbs extra virgin olive oil
2 brown onions, thinly sliced
  into rounds
1 tbs finely grated fresh ginger
2 garlic cloves, crushed
60g (¼ cup) Madras curry paste,
  or korma curry paste
¼ cauliflower, chopped
½ pumpkin, chopped
2 handfuls green beans, chopped
400g (2 cups) basmati rice
2 tbs currants
1L (4 cups) water
35g (⅓ cup) flaked almonds, toasted
½ cup fresh coriander sprigs
Natural yoghurt, to serve

1 Heat the butter and 1 tbs oil in a large heavy-based saucepan over medium-low heat. Add the onion, ginger and garlic. Cook, stirring occasionally, for 12 minutes or until softened and golden. Season. Transfer to a bowl. Set aside.

2 Heat the remaining oil in the pan over medium heat. Add the curry paste. Cook, stirring, for 1-2 minutes or until aromatic. Set aside 2 tbs onion mixture. Add the vegetables, rice, currants and remaining onion mixture. Cook, stirring, for 1 minute or until well combined. Add water and bring to the boil. Reduce heat to low. Cook, covered, for 10 minutes or until the rice and vegetables are tender. Stand, covered, for 10 minutes. Fluff mixture with a fork to separate.

3 Sprinkle biryani with the nuts, coriander and reserved onion mixture. Serve topped with a dollop of yoghurt.

**COOK'S NOTE**

You can use any mix of vegetables for this recipe. You will need a total of 6 cups.

## NUTRITION (PER SERVE)

| CALS | FAT | SAT FAT | PROTEIN | CARBS |
|------|-----|---------|---------|-------|
| 482 | 16.9g | 4g | 12.2g | 66.2g |

● EASY  ● FAMILY-FRIENDLY  ● GLUTEN FREE  ● LOW CAL  ○ QUICK  ○ VEGAN

482
cals

★★★★★

*Great meal. Followed the recipe exactly, but I imagine you could use other vegetables, too. Will add this to the weeknight regular list. Love that you only need one pot.* **LUTAJ**

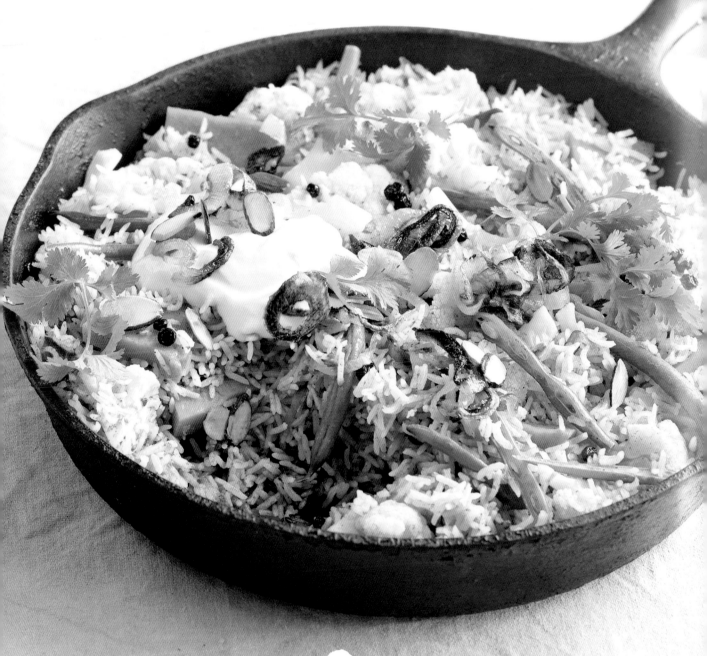

# SLOW COOKER EGGPLANT

# PARMIGIANA

The possibilities in the slow cooker are truly endless! Make this fall-apart tender eggplant parmigiana for dinner and everyone will think you slaved away!

**SERVES** 4  **PREP** 20 mins (+ standing & cooling)  **COOK** 2 hours 40 mins

2 (about 280g each) small eggplants
2 tsp salt
60ml (¼ cup) vegetable stock
400g jar Napoletana pasta sauce
2 tbs olive oil
2 garlic cloves, crushed
40g (⅔ cup) panko breadcrumbs
40g (½ cup) finely grated parmesan
250g piece mozzarella, cut into
   eight 5mm thick slices
Fresh basil leaves, to serve

1. Slice the eggplants in half lengthways. Use a small sharp knife to score the flesh crossways, about 1.5cm apart, leaving skin intact. Sprinkle with salt. Set aside for 20 minutes. Rinse off salt. Gently squeeze out excess liquid.

2. Combine the stock and 185ml (¾ cup) pasta sauce in a jug. Pour into a 5L slow cooker and evenly spread over the base. Arrange the eggplant halves, cut-side up, on top of the sauce. Spread remaining pasta sauce over the eggplant. Cover and cook on High for 2½ hours.

3. Meanwhile, heat the oil in a large frying pan over medium heat. Add the garlic. Cook for 30 seconds or until aromatic. Add the panko. Cook, stirring, for 4 minutes or until golden. Transfer to a large bowl and set aside for 10 minutes to cool slightly. Add the parmesan and toss to combine.

4. Arrange 2 slices mozzarella on top of each eggplant. Fold a clean tea towel in half and place over the slow cooker. Cover and cook on High for 10 minutes or until cheese has melted.

5. Use a large flat spoon or spatula to carefully transfer the eggplant to serving plates. Drizzle sauce around eggplant and spoon panko mixture on top. Scatter over basil leaves, to serve.

## NUTRITION (PER SERVE)

| CALS | FAT | SAT FAT | PROTEIN | CARBS |
|------|-----|---------|---------|-------|
| 486 | 33.7g | 14.1g | 26.5g | 17.2g |

● EASY  ● FAMILY-FRIENDLY  ○ GLUTEN FREE  ● LOW CAL  ○ QUICK  ○ VEGAN

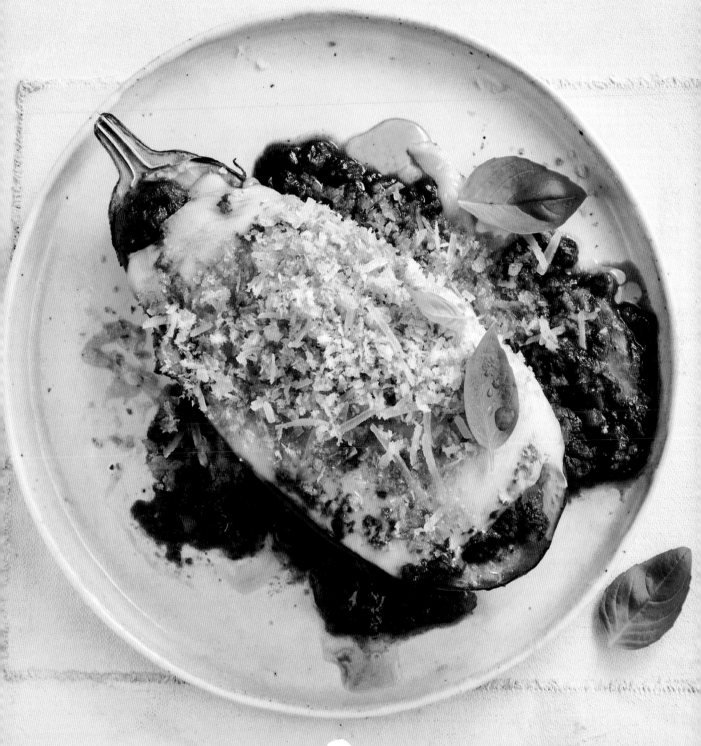

★ ★ ★ ★ ★ *Delicious.* **RACHB78**

486
cals

# HEALTHY TUSCAN BREAD SOUP

Also known as ribollita, this famous Tuscan bread soup makes for a healthy vegetarian dinner. Our version is made in the slow cooker, so it's super easy.

**SERVES** 4  **PREP** 20 mins  **COOK** 4 hours 40 mins

2 tsp olive oil
1 brown onion, finely chopped
2 carrots, peeled, chopped
2 celery sticks, trimmed, chopped
2 garlic cloves, crushed
1 tsp fennel seeds
Pinch of dried chilli flakes
400g can crushed tomatoes
400g can cannellini beans,
    drained, rinsed
1L (4 cups) vegetable stock
Bouquet garni (4 fresh or dried bay
    leaves, 4 fresh sprigs thyme,
    2 fresh sprigs rosemary)
200g cavolo nero (Tuscan cabbage),
    stem removed, leaves shredded
2 thick slices Italian bread
    (pane di casa), lightly toasted,
    torn into chunks
40g (½ cup) finely grated parmesan,
    plus extra, shaved, to serve
1 lemon, rind finely grated, juiced
Finely chopped continental parsley,
    to serve

1 Set a 5L slow cooker to Browning (see note). Add the oil. When oil is hot, add the onion, carrot and celery. Cook, stirring, for 5 minutes or until onion is softened. Add the garlic, fennel and chilli. Cook, stirring, for 1 minute. Add the tomato, beans, stock and bouquet garni. Season. Change slow cooker setting to High. Cover and cook for 3-4 hours or until vegetables are almost tender.

2 Stir in covolo nero, bread and parmesan. Cover and cook on High for 30 minutes or until soup has thickened slightly. Stir in lemon juice, to taste. Serve topped with parsley, lemon rind and extra parmesan.

## NUTRITION (PER SERVE)

| CALS | FAT | SAT FAT | PROTEIN | CARBS |
|------|-----|---------|---------|-------|
| 260  | 8g  | 3.5g    | 14g     | 26.5g |

**COOK'S NOTE**

If your slow cooker doesn't have a browning function, simply fry the vegetables in a frying pan, then transfer to the slow cooker and continue with step 1.

● EASY  ● FAMILY-FRIENDLY  ○ GLUTEN FREE  ● LOW CAL  ○ QUICK  ○ VEGAN

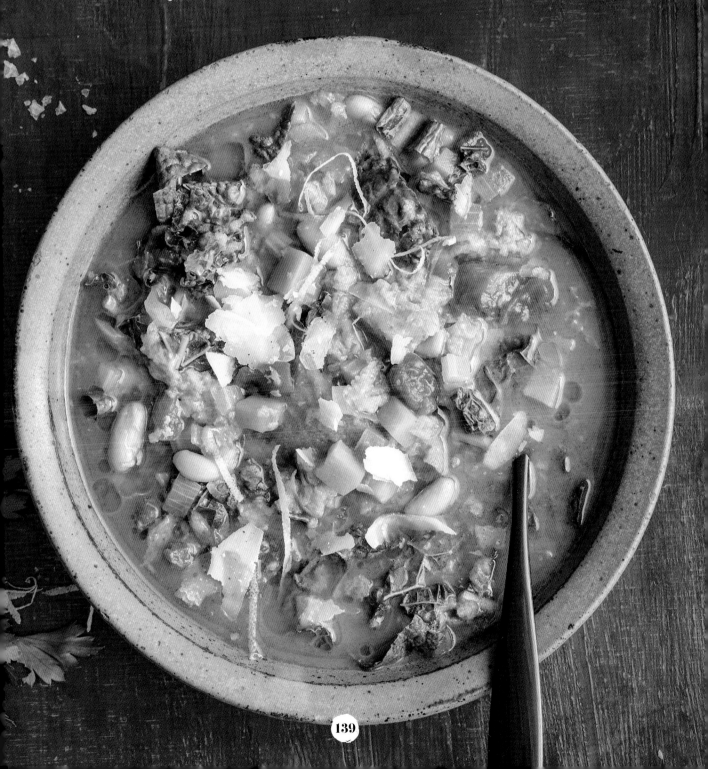

★ ★ ★ ★ ★
Delicious soup. I just make it on the cooktop.
The fennel and lemon add a real zing. **ALLEYCAT1511**

260
*cals*

# MEDITERRANEAN VEGETABLE

# WELLINGTON

With decorated buttery puff pastry and a vibrant Mediterranean-inspired filling, this vegetarian main looks as impressive as it tastes.

**SERVES** 8  **PREP** 30 mins (+ cooling & chilling) **COOK** 45 mins

2 tbs extra virgin olive oil
1 red onion, finely chopped
3 garlic cloves, crushed
1 large eggplant, cut into
   1.5cm pieces
2 zucchini, finely chopped
310g jar roasted pepper strips,
   drained well, coarsely chopped
80g (½ cup) drained sun-dried
   tomatoes, finely chopped
2 tbs finely chopped fresh
   continental parsley leaves
¼ cup finely chopped fresh
   basil leaves
240g (1 cup) fresh ricotta
2 tbs finely chopped pitted
   Sicilian olives
2 eggs, lightly beaten
5 sheets frozen butter puff pastry,
   just thawed
Steamed greens, to serve

**1** Heat the oil in a frying pan over medium-high heat. Add onion, garlic and eggplant. Cover. Cook, stirring occasionally, for 6 minutes or until eggplant softens. Stir through zucchini. Transfer to a tray. Place in the fridge for 15 minutes to cool. Transfer to a bowl. Add peppers, tomato, parsley, basil, ricotta, olive and half the egg. Season. Stir to combine.

**2** Preheat oven to 220°C/200°C fan forced. Line a large baking tray with baking paper. Place 2 sheets of pastry, side-by-side, slightly overlapping, on the prepared tray. Press overlapping edge to secure. Spoon ricotta mixture onto centre. Shape into a 30cm-long log.

**3** Place another 2 pastry sheets, side-by-side, slightly overlapping, on a work surface. Press overlapping edge to secure. Carefully place on top of ricotta log, pressing around edges of log to enclose. Trim excess pastry. Roll and pinch edges together to seal. Cut 3cm- and 5cm-long leaves from remaining pastry sheet. Brush pastry log with egg. Using picture as a guide, arrange leaves on top. Brush leaves with remaining egg. Season. Place in the fridge for 30 minutes to firm up a little.

**4** Bake for 35-40 minutes or until pastry is golden. Stand on tray for 5 minutes. Transfer to a serving board. Slice and serve with steamed greens.

## NUTRITION (PER SERVE)

| CALS | FAT | SAT FAT | PROTEIN | CARBS |
|------|------|---------|---------|-------|
| 541 | 30.2g | 16.7g | 14.7g | 47.5g |

○ EASY  ● FAMILY-FRIENDLY  ○ GLUTEN FREE  ● LOW CAL  ○ QUICK  ○ VEGAN

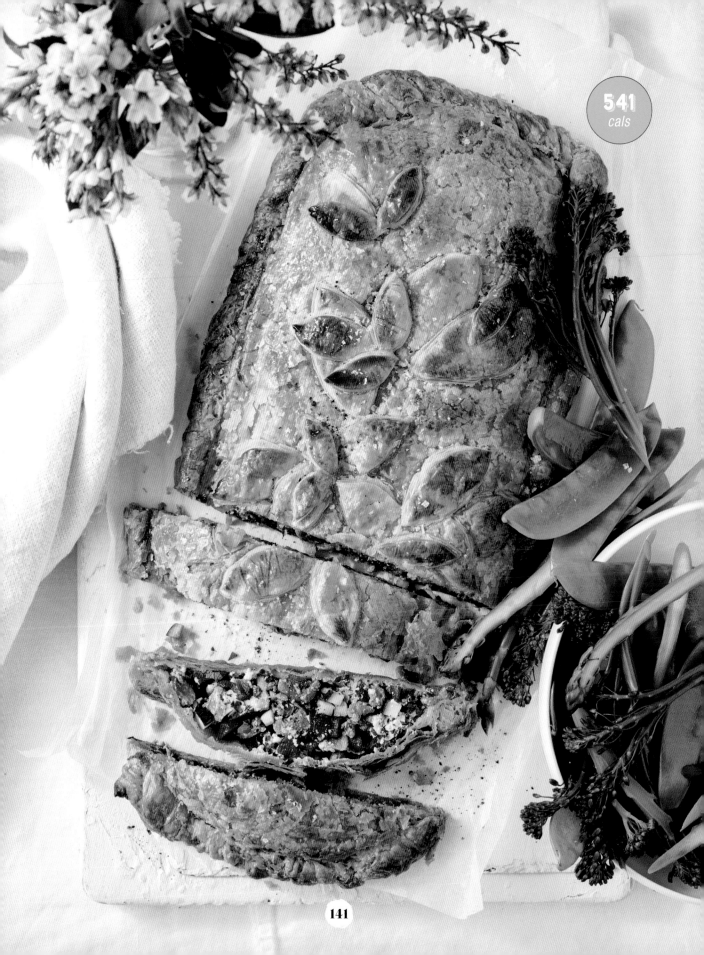

541
cals

# LASAGNE WITH ZUCCHINI LATTICE

Get your veg on with this stunning lasagne that will fill up even the most die-hard meat-eater. The lovely latticework makes it dinner-party worthy.

**SERVES** 8   **PREP** 30 mins (+ standing)   **COOK** 1 hour

20g butter
1 tbs extra virgin olive oil
1 leek, trimmed, thinly sliced
3 large garlic cloves
3 bunches English spinach, trimmed,
   washed, chopped
3 medium zucchini, coarsely grated,
   plus 3 large zucchini, thinly sliced
1 bunch fresh basil, chopped
480g (2 cups) fresh ricotta
300ml tub light thickened cream
70g (1 cup) finely grated parmesan
1 tsp finely grated lemon rind
Pinch of nutmeg
2 eggs, lightly beaten
250ml (1 cup) tomato pasta sauce
200g (2 cups) pre-grated four
   cheese melt
9 dried lasagne sheets
55g (⅓ cup) pine nuts
Mixed baby salad leaves,
   to serve

1 Preheat the oven to 200°C/180°C fan forced. Lightly grease a 20 x 26cm (base measurement) baking dish.

2 Heat butter and oil in a large frying pan over medium-high heat until foaming. Add the leek and garlic. Reduce heat to medium-low. Cook, stirring often, for 5 minutes or until leek has softened. Add the spinach and grated zucchini. Increase heat to high. Cook, stirring often, for 5 minutes or until spinach wilts and any excess liquid has evaporated. Stir in the basil. Season well.

3 Whisk the ricotta, cream, parmesan, lemon rind, nutmeg and egg in a bowl until combined. Season well.

4 Spread one-third of the pasta sauce over base of the prepared dish. Sprinkle with a little cheese. Top with a layer of pasta (break to fit as necessary), one-quarter of the ricotta mixture and one-third of the spinach mixture. Repeat with half the remaining pasta sauce, one-third of the remaining cheese, one-third of the remaining ricotta mixture and half the remaining spinach mixture. Top with the remaining pasta sauce, half the remaining cheese, half the remaining ricotta mixture and the remaining spinach mixture. Cover with remaining ricotta mixture. Sprinkle with almost all the remaining cheese.

5 Layer the zucchini slices in a lattice pattern over the top of the lasagne. Sprinkle with the remaining cheese.

6 Bake lasagne for 40 minutes or until starting to brown. Sprinkle with pine nuts. Bake for 5-10 minutes or until pine nuts are golden. Set aside for 10 minutes to rest. Serve with baby salad leaves.

## NUTRITION (PER SERVE)

| CALS | FAT | SAT FAT | PROTEIN | CARBS |
|------|------|---------|---------|-------|
| 574 | 38.1g | 12.7g | 25.9g | 26.3g |

○ EASY   ● FAMILY-FRIENDLY   ○ GLUTEN FREE   ● LOW CAL   ○ QUICK   ○ VEGAN

★★★★★

*Sometimes lasagne can be a bit heavy – this one isn't – it's refreshingly light and you can eat a big slab without feeling bloated :) I was glad I did the lattice, worth the bit of effort as it stayed nicely crunchy.* **MAREEO**

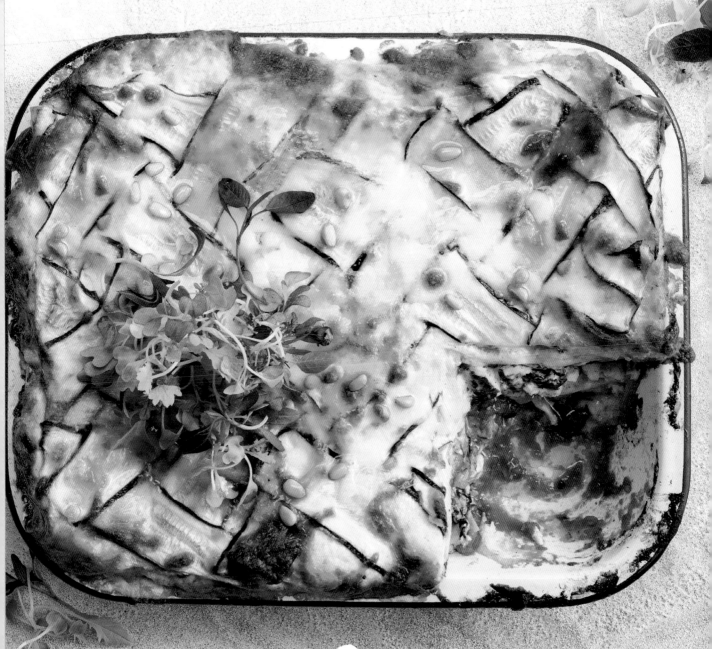

# RISOTTO
# PRIMAVERA

This light and fresh risotto primavera is jam-packed with seasonal offerings. Feel free to swap the veg for other types you like, to really make it yours.

**SERVES** 4  **PREP** 10 mins  **COOK** 45 mins

1L (4 cups) vegetable stock
250ml (1 cup) water
1 bunch baby (Dutch) carrots, trimmed, peeled
1 bunch asparagus, trimmed, cut into 4cm lengths
150g sugar snap peas, trimmed
4 spring onions (globe onions)
1½ tbs olive oil
1 small brown onion, finely chopped
330g (1½ cups) arborio rice
125ml (½ cup) dry white wine
70g (1 cup) finely grated parmesan
½ cup coarsely chopped fresh basil leaves

1 Place stock and water in a large saucepan over high heat. Cover. Bring to the boil. Add carrots. Reduce heat to medium. Simmer, covered, for 2 minutes. Add asparagus and peas. Simmer, covered, for 2 minutes or until just tender. Use a slotted spoon to transfer vegetables to a bowl. Cover to keep warm. Remove stock from heat. Cover to keep warm.

2 Trim tops and roots of spring onions. Cut bulb into quarters. Heat the oil in a large saucepan over medium-high heat. Add spring onion. Cook, covered, stirring occasionally for 5 minutes or until golden and just tender. Transfer to the vegetables in the bowl. Cover to keep warm.

3 Add brown onion to pan. Cook, stirring, for 5 minutes or until softened. Add rice. Cook, stirring, for 1 minute. Add wine. Simmer for 30 seconds. Add 80ml (⅓ cup) stock to rice mixture. Cook, stirring, until stock is absorbed. Repeat with remaining stock, 80ml (⅓ cup) at a time, until liquid is absorbed and rice is tender.

4 Add vegetables and 60g (¾ cup) parmesan to pan. Stir. Remove from heat. Stand, covered, for 2 minutes or until vegetables are heated through and cheese has melted. Season. Stir in basil and top with remaining parmesan. Serve.

## NUTRITION (PER SERVE)

| CALS | FAT | SAT FAT | PROTEIN | CARBS |
| --- | --- | --- | --- | --- |
| 505 | 16g | 6g | 18g | 67g |

★★★★★

*What I really liked was the freshness and sweet crunchiness of the asparagus and baby carrots. A great vegetarian meal.* **CHOCOLATE POODLE**

○ EASY  ● FAMILY-FRIENDLY  ○ GLUTEN FREE  ● LOW CAL  ○ QUICK  ○ VEGAN

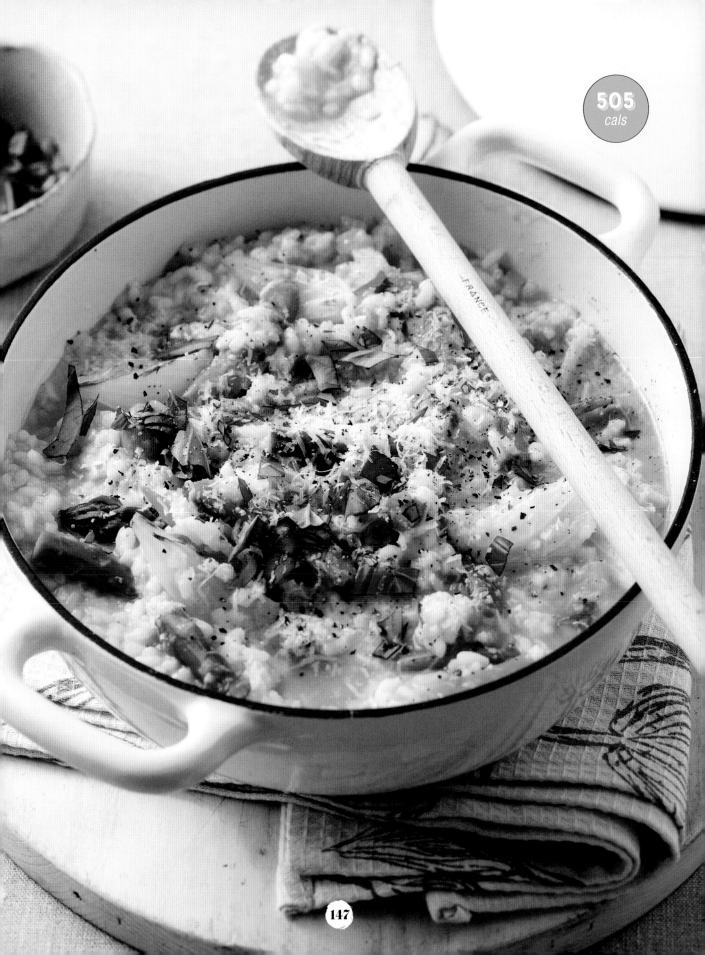

# QUICK SUPER-GREEN
# MEE GORENG

Packed with six types of veg, this tasty Asian noodle stir-fry is on the table in just 25 minutes. Perfect for keeping healthy on busy nights.

**SERVES** 4 **PREP** 15 mins **COOK** 10 mins

200g dried egg noodles
1 tbs peanut oil
1 brown onion, thinly sliced
1 bunch broccolini, trimmed, halved
  lengthways and crossways
1 zucchini, cut into 2cm pieces
100g sugar snap peas, trimmed
2 garlic cloves, crushed
2cm-piece fresh ginger, peeled,
  finely grated
1 bunch baby pak choy, halved
  lengthways
¼ wombok, coarsely chopped
2 tbs kecap manis
1½ tbs soy sauce
1 tbs lime juice
60g (⅓ cup) dry-roasted almonds,
  chopped
Sliced small red chilli, to serve

1 Cook noodles in a large saucepan of boiling salted water, following packet directions. Drain.

2 Meanwhile, heat a wok over medium-high heat. Add oil. Swirl to coat. Add onion. Cook, stirring, for 2 minutes or until softened. Add broccolini, zucchini, peas, garlic and ginger. Cook, stirring, for 2 minutes or until the broccolini is tender.

3 Add noodles, pak choy, wombok, sauces and lime juice to the pan. Cook, stirring, for 1-2 minutes or until heated through. Serve sprinkled with almond and chilli.

## NUTRITION (PER SERVE)

| CALS | FAT | SAT FAT | PROTEIN | CARBS |
|------|-----|---------|---------|-------|
| 364 | 11.7g | 1.5g | 14.3g | 46.4g |

### COOK'S NOTE

If you want to ramp up the protein, cook a couple of eggs omelette-style, chop, then stir through noodles at the end to heat through.

★★★★★

*We love a vegetarian dish and this one will leave you feeling light and healthy!* **SARAH.DEJONG**

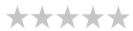

● EASY  ● FAMILY-FRIENDLY  ○ GLUTEN FREE  ● LOW CAL  ● QUICK  ○ VEGAN

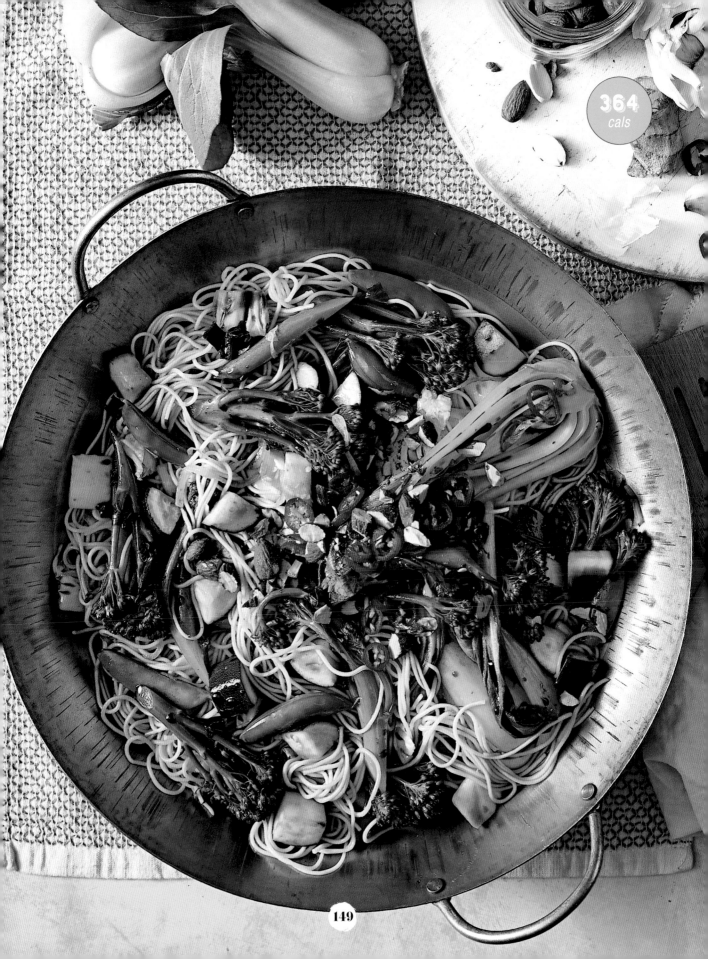

364
cals

# MUSHROOM STROGANOFF
## PASTA BAKE

While it's good to know this creamy strog bake is made with three serves of veg, all big and small kids need to know is that it tastes out of this world!

**SERVES** 6  **PREP** 15 mins  **COOK** 30 mins

375g dried penne pasta
2 tbs extra virgin olive oil
200g portobello mushrooms, thickly sliced
200g Swiss brown mushrooms, halved
200g button mushrooms, halved
20g butter
1 brown onion, thinly sliced
2 garlic cloves, crushed
125ml (½ cup) dry white wine
2 tbs tomato paste
300g tub light sour cream
1 tsp smoked paprika
120g baby spinach
¼ cup chopped fresh tarragon
¾ cup grated pizza cheese
Fresh continental parsley leaves, to serve

1 Cook pasta in a large saucepan of salted boiling water following packet directions or until al dente. Drain, reserving 80ml (⅓ cup) cooking liquid. Return pasta to pan. Cover to keep warm.

2 Meanwhile, heat 1 tbs oil in a large frying pan over high heat. Cook half of all mushrooms, tossing occasionally, for 4-5 minutes or until golden. Transfer to a plate. Repeat with remaining oil and mushrooms. Set aside.

3 Reduce heat to medium-low. Melt butter in the pan. Add onion. Cook, stirring, for 3-4 minutes or until softened. Add garlic. Cook for 30 seconds or until aromatic. Add wine. Simmer for 2 minutes or until reduced by half. Stir in tomato paste, sour cream and paprika. Simmer for 2-3 minutes or until thickened slightly. Season. Return mushrooms to pan with spinach and tarragon. Cook for 2 minutes or until heated through and spinach has just wilted.

4 Preheat oven grill on high. Add mushroom mixture and reserved cooking liquid to pasta. Toss to combine. Spoon into a 2L (8-cup) ovenproof dish. Sprinkle with the cheese. Grill for 4-5 minutes or until cheese is golden and melted. Sprinkle with parsley, to serve.

## NUTRITION (PER SERVE)

| CALS | FAT | SAT FAT | PROTEIN | CARBS |
|------|-----|---------|---------|-------|
| 520 | 23.8g | 11.7g | 16.9g | 52.1g |

★★★★★ *This pasta bake is delicious! I'm trying to eat less meat and didn't even miss it in this. Will be making this regularly.* **LAURENMCD**

● EASY  ● FAMILY-FRIENDLY  ○ GLUTEN FREE  ● LOW CAL  ○ QUICK  ○ VEGAN

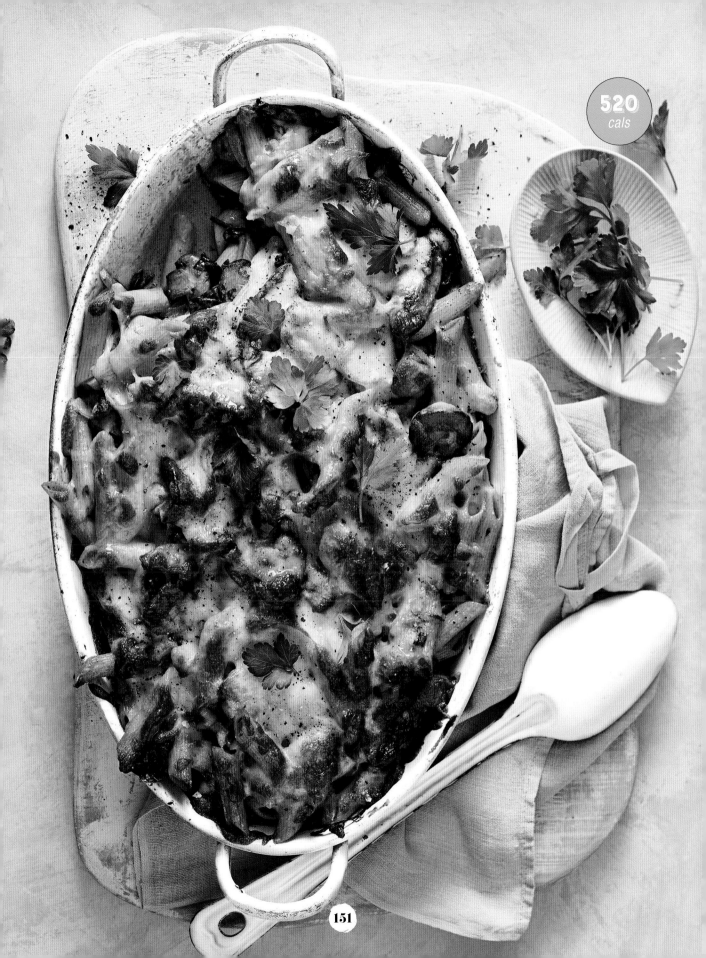

520
cals

# NORTH INDIAN PANEER CURRY

Low-cal, gluten-free and packed with lean protein, this hearty vegie curry, with spice and all things nice, truly is a one-pot wonder.

**SERVES** 4 **PREP** 15 mins **COOK** 45 mins

2 tsp macadamia oil
200g paneer cheese, drained, cut into 2cm pieces
1 large red onion, finely chopped
1 tbs finely grated fresh ginger
2 garlic cloves, crushed
1 long fresh green chilli, deseeded, finely chopped, plus extra, sliced, to serve
2 tsp ground cumin
2 tsp ground coriander
1 tsp ground turmeric
2 tbs no-added-salt tomato paste
4 large tomatoes, peeled, chopped
250ml (1 cup) water
200g cauliflower, cut into small florets
150g (1 cup) frozen peas
270g (2 cups) steamed brown rice
Fresh coriander leaves, to serve

1 Heat half the oil in a large saucepan over medium-high heat. Cook the paneer, in batches, for 1-2 minutes each side or until golden. Transfer to a plate.

2 Reduce heat to medium. Add remaining oil and onion. Cook, stirring, for 3-4 minutes or until softened. Add ginger, garlic, chilli, cumin, ground coriander and turmeric. Cook, stirring, for 3-4 minutes or until aromatic. Stir in the tomato paste and cook for 1 minute. Add tomato and water. Bring to the boil. Reduce heat to medium-low. Cover and simmer for 15 minutes.

3 Add the cauliflower. Simmer, covered, for 5 minutes or until tender. Add the peas and paneer, and simmer for 3-4 minutes or until peas are tender. Serve on brown rice, sprinkled with extra chilli and coriander.

## COOK'S NOTE

Paneer is a firm cheese, similar to firm ricotta or feta (though not as salty). You'll find it near the feta at the supermarket.

## NUTRITION (PER SERVE)

| CALS | FAT | SAT FAT | PROTEIN | CARBS |
| --- | --- | --- | --- | --- |
| 370 | 10.2g | 2.6g | 27.4g | 29.1g |

● EASY  ○ FAMILY-FRIENDLY  ● GLUTEN FREE  ● LOW CAL  ○ QUICK  ○ VEGAN

364
*cals*

★ ★ ★ ★ ★

*I love that this dish is healthy, but it doesn't sceimp on flavoue. A good recipe to keep on hand.* **CHARLIEDINNER**

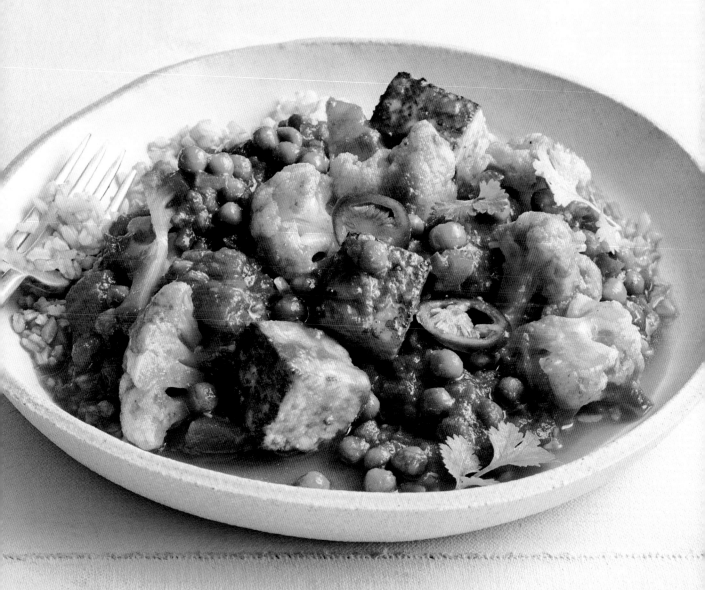

# STUFFED BUCKWHEAT CRESPELLE

These gluten-free Italian-style crepes are filled to the brim with ricotta, spinach and sun-dried tomatoes, then drizzled in tangy passata.

**SERVES** 6 **PREP** 30 mins (+ standing) **COOK** 1 hour 5 mins

2 tsp extra virgin olive oil
280g pkt baby spinach leaves
700g fresh ricotta, crumbled
100g sun-dried tomatoes,
  finely chopped
½ cup fresh basil leaves,
  finely chopped
2 tbs finely chopped fresh chives
1 lemon, rind finely grated
40g (½ cup) finely grated pecorino
250ml (1 cup) tomato passata

### CRESPELLE
150g (1 cup) buckwheat flour
3 eggs, lightly beaten
250ml (1 cup) reduced-fat milk
20g butter, melted, cooled, plus
  20g extra butter, chopped, to fry
60ml (¼ cup) water

1 Heat half the oil in a large frying pan over high heat. Add half the spinach. Cook, stirring, for 1-2 minutes or until just wilted. Transfer to a bowl. Repeat with remaining oil and spinach. Cool completely. Squeeze excess liquid from spinach.

2 To make the crespelle, place the flour in a bowl. Use a wooden spoon to stir in the egg until well combined. Stir in 60ml (¼ cup) milk until smooth. Stir in the remaining milk. Slowly stir in butter. Set aside for 10 minutes. Strain through a sieve into a bowl. Stir in water until the consistency of pouring cream.

3 Heat a 20cm (base) non-stick frying pan over low heat. Add a little butter. Swirl to coat pan. Pour in just under ¼ cup batter. Tilt to cover base. Cook for 1-2 minutes or until edges start to curl. Turn over and cook for a further 1-2 minutes or until golden. Transfer to a plate and cover with a clean tea towel to keep warm. Repeat with butter and batter to make 12 crespelle.

4 Preheat oven to 200°C/180°C fan forced. Lightly grease a large baking dish. Combine the ricotta, tomato, basil, chives, lemon rind, spinach and half the cheese in a bowl. Season well.

5 Place 1 crespelle on a clean work surface. Spread half with some ricotta mixture. Fold in half, then half again, to form a curved triangle. Repeat with remaining crespelle and ricotta mixture.

6 Pour two-thirds of the passata into the prepared dish. Arrange crespelle on top in rows. Drizzle remaining passata over crespelle. Sprinkle with remaining pecorino. Bake for 12 minutes or until golden. Serve.

## NUTRITION (PER SERVE)

| CALS | FAT | SAT FAT | PROTEIN | CARBS |
|------|-----|---------|---------|-------|
| 450 | 22.5g | 12.1g | 26.8g | 39.9g |

○ EASY  ● FAMILY-FRIENDLY  ● GLUTEN FREE  ● LOW CAL  ○ QUICK  ○ VEGAN

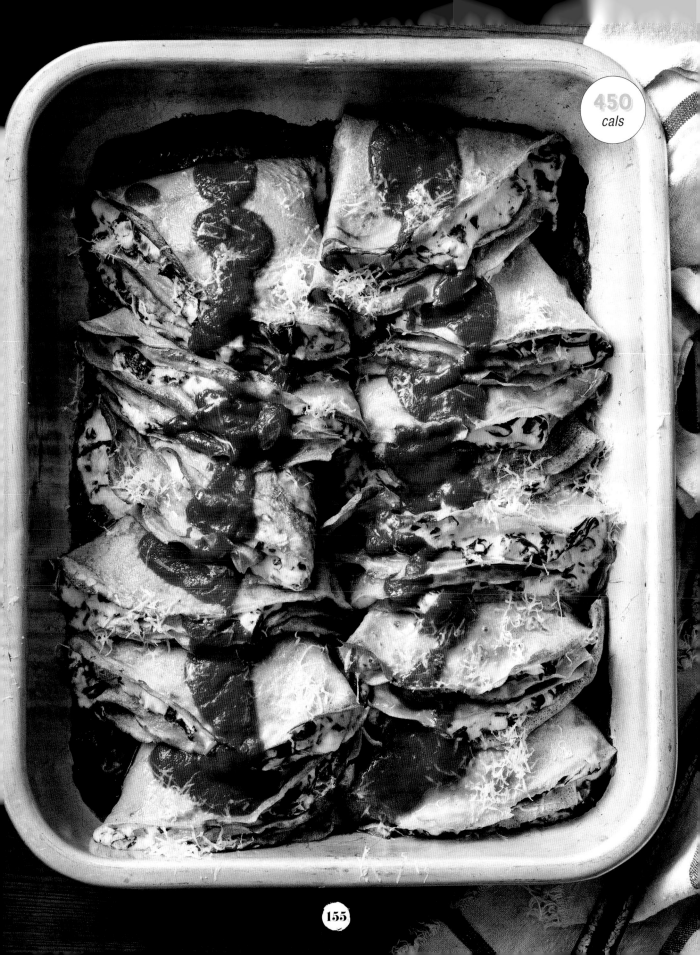

450 cals

155

# JAPANESE TOFU KATSU

This classic Japanese curry gets a vego twist by switching out the chicken for tofu. Think of the nori on top as a sprinkle of vitamin C.

**SERVES** 6 **PREP** 20 mins **COOK** 25 mins

1 tbs vegetable oil, plus extra, to shallow-fry
1 small brown onion, thinly sliced
2 tsp finely grated fresh ginger
2 garlic cloves, crushed
1 small red apple, grated
92g pkt golden curry sauce mix
625ml (2½ cups) vegetable stock
2 carrots, peeled, halved, thinly sliced diagonally
150g shiitake mushrooms, halved if large
500g firm tofu
75g (½ cup) plain flour
1 egg, lightly beaten
5g pkt roasted seaweed snacks
50g (1 cup) panko breadcrumbs
Steamed rice, thinly sliced radish and thinly sliced cucumber, to serve

1 Heat the oil in a large saucepan over medium heat. Add the onion and cook, stirring, for 2-3 minutes or until softened. Add the ginger and garlic. Cook, stirring, for 1 minute or until aromatic. Add the apple and curry sauce mix. Stir for 30 seconds. Add stock and carrot. Bring to the boil. Reduce heat to low and simmer, covered, for 5 minutes. Add the mushrooms. Cook, uncovered, for 10 minutes or until all vegies are tender.

2 Meanwhile, cut the tofu into 8 large slices. Place the flour on a plate and season. Place the egg and 1 tbs water in a shallow bowl. Whisk to combine. Finely chop half the seaweed and combine with the breadcrumbs on a separate plate. Dip the tofu in the flour and shake off any excess. Dip in egg, then breadcrumb mixture, pressing firmly to coat.

3 Add enough oil to a large frying pan to come 1cm up the side. Heat over medium-high heat. Cook tofu, in 2 batches, for 2-3 minutes each side or until crisp. Transfer to a plate lined with paper towel to drain. Thickly slice tofu.

4 Serve the tofu and vegie curry over steamed rice and topped with radish and cucumber. Thinly slice the remaining seaweed and sprinkle on top, to serve.

## COOK'S NOTE

You can make the vegie curry and fry the tofu up to 2 days ahead. Store in separate airtight containers in the fridge. Heat the curry on the stovetop and the tofu in the oven until crisp. Continue with step 4, to serve.

## NUTRITION (PER SERVE)

| CALS | FAT | SAT FAT | PROTEIN | CARBS |
|------|------|---------|---------|-------|
| 448 | 20.7g | 4g | 17.3g | 43.3g |

○ EASY ○ FAMILY-FRIENDLY ○ GLUTEN FREE ● LOW CAL ○ QUICK ○ VEGAN

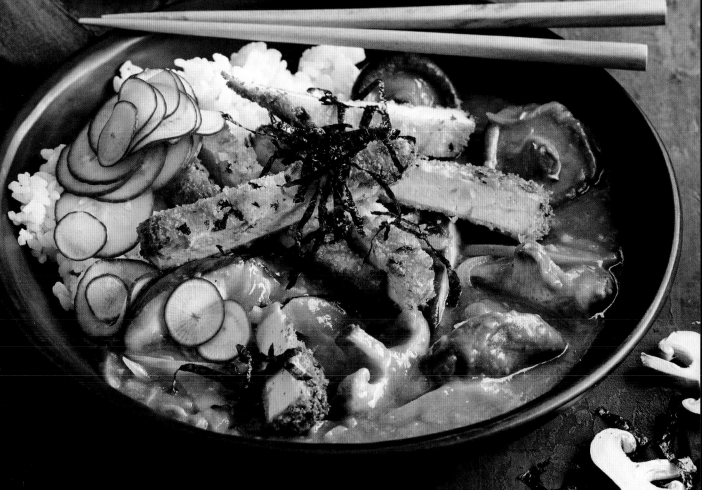

448 cals

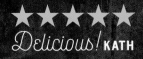

★★★★★
Delicious! KATH

# PUMPKIN
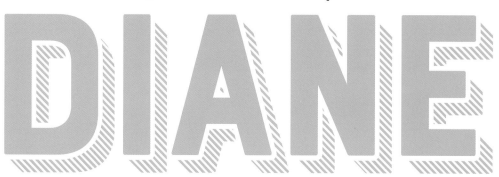
# DIANE

We've taken a family favourite dinner and put a healthier, vegetarian spin on it – introducing pumpkin Diane! You'll love it as much as we do.

**SERVES** 4  **PREP** 15 mins  **COOK** 35 mins

800g kent pumpkin, deseeded, cut into 2cm-thick wedges

200g button mushrooms, halved

1 tbs extra virgin olive oil

1 large red onion, halved, thickly sliced

3 garlic cloves, crushed

400g can gluten-free lentils, rinsed, drained

¼ cup chopped fresh herbs (such as chives, parsley)

1 French shallot, finely chopped

125ml (½ cup) light cream for cooking

80ml (⅓ cup) salt-reduced gluten-free vegetable stock

2 tbs gluten-free Worcestershire sauce

1 tbs Dijon mustard

**1** Preheat oven to 200°C/180°C fan forced. Line a large baking tray with baking paper. Arrange the pumpkin on the prepared tray in a single layer. Lightly spray with oil. Bake for 15 minutes. Add mushroom and spray with a little more oil. Bake for 15-20 minutes or until vegies are golden and tender.

**2** Meanwhile, heat 2 tsp oil in a large non-stick frying pan over medium heat. Cook onion, stirring, for 6 minutes or until softened. Add one-third of the garlic. Cook, stirring for 1 minute or until aromatic. Stir in the lentils. Cook, stirring, for 2 minutes or until warmed through. Season. Stir in the herbs. Remove from the heat and cover to keep warm.

**3** Heat remaining oil in a small saucepan over medium heat. Cook shallot, stirring, for 3 minutes or until softened. Add the remaining garlic. Cook, stirring, for 1 minute or until aromatic. Whisk in cream, stock, Worcestershire and mustard until well combined. Simmer gently for 2-3 minutes or until slightly thickened. Scatter vegies with lentil mixture. Drizzle with sauce, to serve.

## NUTRITION (PER SERVE)

| CALS | FAT | SAT FAT | PROTEIN | CARBS |
|------|-----|---------|---------|-------|
| 273 | 14g | 4.9g | 9.1g | 22.3g |

★★★★★

*Amazing. Really tasty and super easy to make.* **LYNHARVEY68**

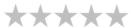

● EASY  ○ FAMILY-FRIENDLY  ● GLUTEN FREE  ● LOW CAL  ○ QUICK  ○ VEGAN

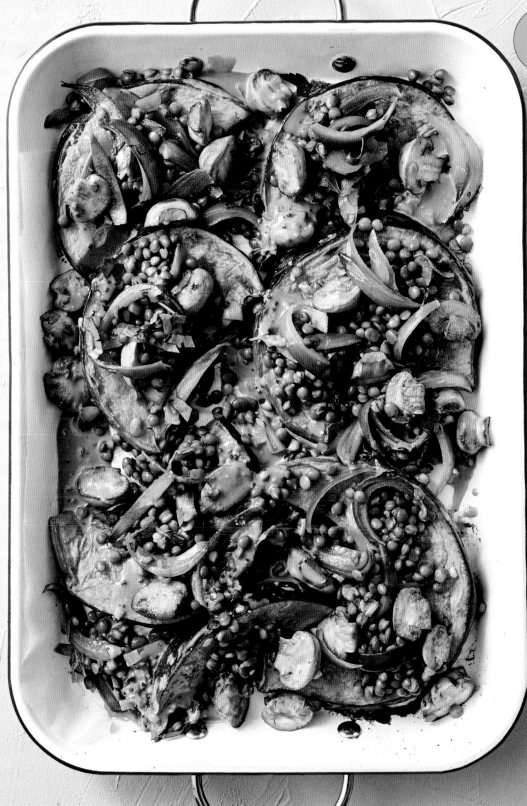

273
cals

# FAST FALAFEL & BLACK RICE
# TABOULI

If you're in a bit of a rush but don't want to compromise on flavour, this super quick and easy lunch or dinner bowl should be on the menu.

**SERVES** 4  **PREP** 15 mins  **COOK** 15 mins

250g pkt microwave black rice
1 small lemon, juiced
1 tbs extra virgin olive oil,
    plus extra, to serve
1 garlic clove, crushed
Large pinch brown sugar
2 bunches fresh mint
1 bunch fresh continental
    parsley leaves
2 truss tomatoes, finely chopped
½ small red onion, finely chopped
150g (1 cup) baby peas, blanched
225g pkt fresh gluten-free falafel
200g tub hummus
Ground cumin, to serve
Natural sliced almonds and mixed
    seeds, toasted, to serve (optional)

1 Cook the rice following packet directions. Transfer to a large bowl. Set aside.

2 Whisk the lemon juice, oil, garlic and sugar in a bowl. Season. Reserve a few small mint sprigs. Chop the remaining mint and parsley, and add to the rice with the tomato, onion and peas. Pour over the lemon dressing and toss to combine. Divide among serving bowls.

3 Heat the falafel following packet directions. Divide the tabouli among serving bowls and top with falafel, dollops of hummus and reserved mint sprigs. Drizzle hummus with extra oil. Sprinkle with cumin, plus the nuts and seeds, if using. Serve.

**COOK'S NOTE**

Assemble the falafels, tabouli and hummus in wraps, if you like, for a convenient lunch.

## NUTRITION (PER SERVE)

| CALS | FAT | SAT FAT | PROTEIN | CARBS |
|------|-----|---------|---------|-------|
| 504 | 27g | 4g | 14g | 44g |

★★★★★

*Delicious, super fresh, fragrant and easy to whip up. Always a winner.* **SHERRIGILCHRIST**

● EASY  ○ FAMILY-FRIENDLY  ● GLUTEN FREE  ● LOW CAL  ● QUICK  ● VEGAN

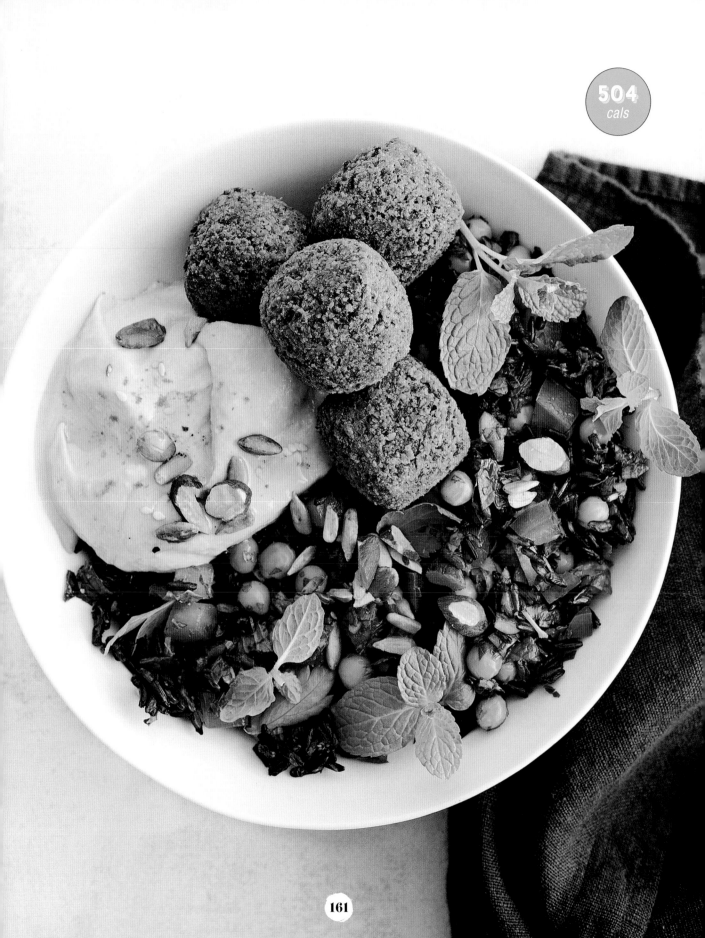

504
*cals*

# EGGPLANT PARMIGIANA LASAGNE

This golden vegetarian bake is heavy on the cheese and comfort, but light on calories. Guaranteed to satisfy the crankiest of carnivores.

**SERVES** 6  **PREP** 20 mins (+ standing)  **COOK** 1 hour 20 mins

3 (about 350g each) eggplant,
  cut into 1cm-thick slices
1 tbs olive oil
1 small brown onion, finely chopped
2 garlic cloves, crushed
700g btl passata
80ml (⅓ cup) water
500g tub smooth ricotta
70g (1 cup) finely grated parmesan
6 fresh lasagne sheets
50g (½ cup) coarsely grated
  mozzarella
Fresh oregano leaves, to serve

1 Preheat oven to 200°C/180°C fan forced. Heat a large frying pan over medium-high heat. Spray the eggplant slices with olive oil. Working in batches, cook the eggplant for 3-4 minutes each side or until soft and golden. Transfer to a plate.

2 Heat the oil in a saucepan over medium heat. Add the onion. Cook, stirring, occasionally, for 4 minutes or until softened. Add the garlic and cook, stirring, for 1 minute or until aromatic. Add the passata. Add the water to the passata bottle, swirl, and pour into the pan. Stir to combine. Bring to the boil. Reduce heat to low and simmer for 5 minutes or until reduced slightly. Season.

3 Combine the ricotta and parmesan in a bowl. Spread one-third of the tomato mixture over the base of a deep 23cm ovenproof dish. Place 2 pasta sheets over the sauce, cutting to fit, as needed. Top with one-third of the eggplant slices. Dot with half the ricotta mixture. Smooth the surface. Repeat with another 2 pasta sheets, half the remaining tomato mixture, half the remaining eggplant and the remaining ricotta mixture. Top with remaining pasta sheets and eggplant. Top with remaining tomato mixture.

4 Cover with foil and bake for 30 minutes. Uncover, sprinkle with mozzarella and bake for 20 minutes or until golden. Stand for 10 minutes. Sprinkle with fresh oregano, to serve.

## NUTRITION (PER SERVE)

| CALS | FAT | SAT FAT | PROTEIN | CARBS |
|------|-----|---------|---------|-------|
| 355 | 22g | 12.1g | 20.9g | 16.4g |

○ EASY  ● FAMILY-FRIENDLY  ○ GLUTEN FREE  ● LOW CAL  ○ QUICK  ○ VEGAN

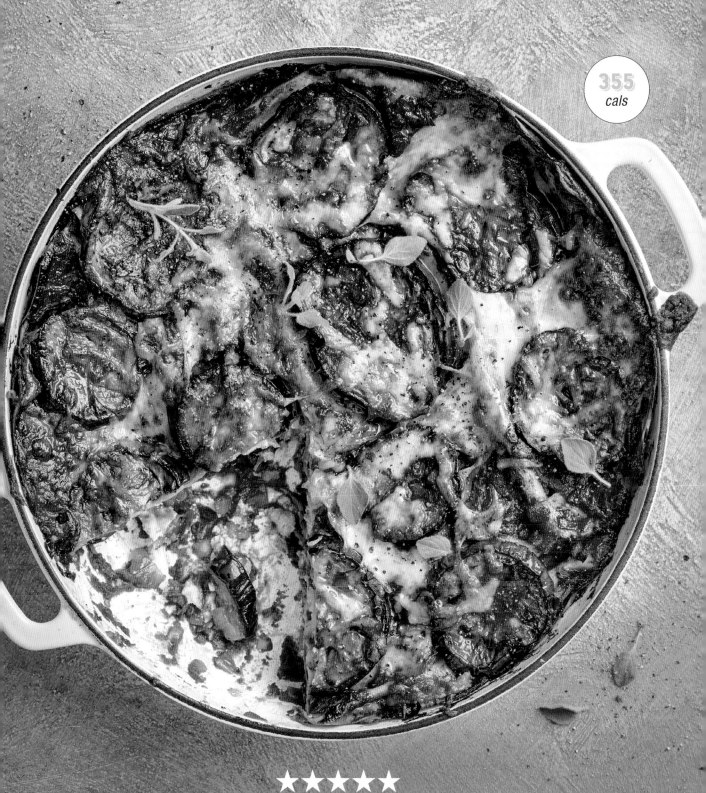

355
cals

★★★★★

Easy and delicious! I love the combination of eggplant and tomato sauce – will definitely be making this lasagne again. ROMMIE

# CRISPY CAESAR
# SALAD

With crispy 'chicken' pieces and a sprinkle of 'bacon' bits, this gorgeously plated plant-based salad will fool even the most loyal of meat-eaters.

**SERVES** 4  **PREP** 20 mins  **COOK** 30 mins

400g pkt vegan 'chicken' nuggets
2 baby cos lettuce, leaves separated
6 qukes (baby cucumbers),
    sliced lengthways
4 radishes, thinly sliced
200g yellow grape tomatoes,
    halved
1 avocado, sliced

**'BACON' BITS**
2 tsp soy sauce
2 tsp maple syrup
1 tsp olive oil
½ tsp smoked paprika
40g (⅔ cup) coconut flakes

**DRESSING**
180g (⅔ cup) natural almond yoghurt
2 tbs tahini
2 tbs fresh lemon juice

1 To make the 'bacon' bits, preheat oven to 150°C/130°C fan forced. Line a large baking tray with baking paper. Combine all the ingredients in a large bowl and toss to coat. Evenly spread over the prepared tray. Bake for 10 minutes or until the coconut flakes are lightly golden. Remove from the oven, toss well and spread out again on the tray. Bake for a further 5 minutes. Set aside to cool (the coconut flakes will be become even more crisp as they cool).

2 Increase oven to 200°C/180°C fan forced. Line a large baking tray with baking paper. Place the nuggets on the prepared tray and bake, turning halfway through cooking, for 10-15 minutes or until golden and cooked through.

3 Meanwhile, to make the dressing, whisk all the ingredients in a jug with 2-3 tbs water. Season with salt. Pour in a little more water to thin the dressing, if necessary.

4 Arrange the lettuce, quke, 'chicken' nuggets, radish, tomato and avocado on a large serving platter or shallow bowl. Dollop with the dressing and season. Sprinkle with the 'bacon' bits, to serve.

## NUTRITION (PER SERVE)

| CALS | FAT | SAT FAT | PROTEIN | CARBS |
| --- | --- | --- | --- | --- |
| 487 | 24.1g | 5.7g | 13.8g | 23.4g |

● EASY  ● FAMILY-FRIENDLY  ○ GLUTEN FREE  ● LOW CAL  ○ QUICK  ● VEGAN

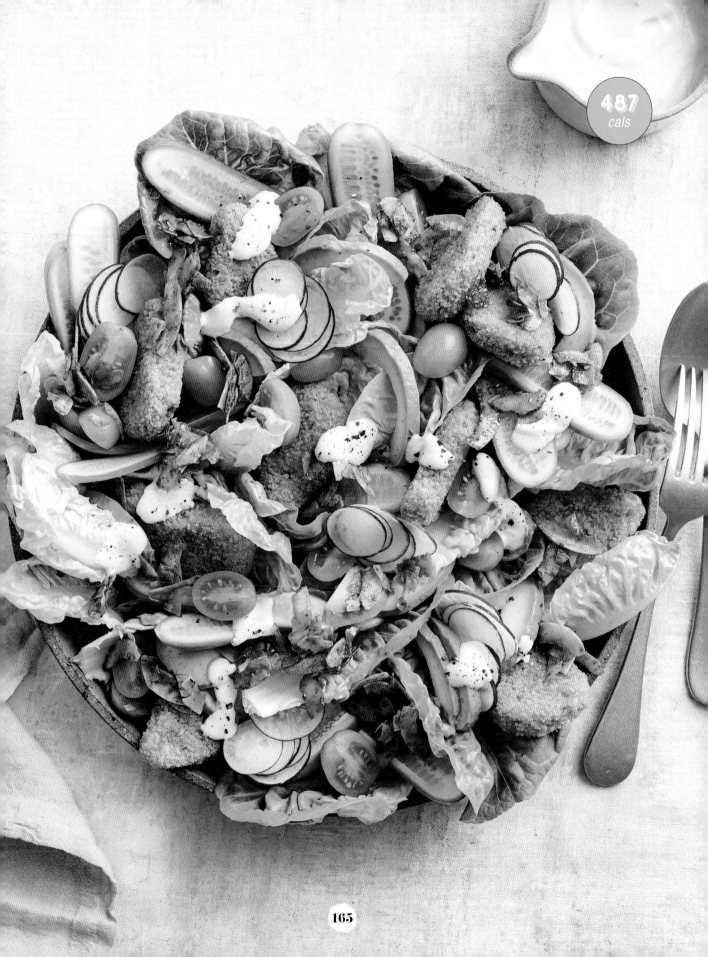

487
cals

# INDIAN-STYLE 'BUTTER' BROCCOLI

Recreate traditional butter chicken with nutrient-dense broccoli and all those wonderful Indian spices. It's a deliciously easy vego alternative.

**SERVES** 4  **PREP** 10 mins  **COOK** 15 mins

400g broccoli, trimmed, cut into small florets

60ml (¼ cup) water, plus extra 80ml (⅓ cup) water

3 cardamom pods, crushed

½ cinnamon stick

80g (⅓ cup) tikka masala curry paste

160ml (⅔ cup) tomato passata

250g haloumi, sliced

80g (⅓ cup) crème fraîche, plus extra, to serve

25g (¼ cup) flaked almonds, toasted

Fresh mint and coriander sprigs, and steamed rice, to serve

**1** Heat a wok over high heat. Spray with oil. Add the broccoli and cook, stirring, for 2 minutes. Add the water and cook, stirring, for 5 minutes or until the water has evaporated and the broccoli is tender-crisp. Transfer to a bowl.

**2** Add the cardamom and cinnamon to the wok. Cook, stirring, for 1 minute or until aromatic. Add the curry paste. Stir for 1 minute or until aromatic. Add the passata and extra water. Simmer for 5 minutes or until reduced slightly.

**3** Meanwhile, heat a large non-stick frying pan over medium heat. Cook the haloumi for 1-2 minutes each side or until golden. Transfer to a plate.

**4** Add the crème fraîche and haloumi to the wok. Cook, stirring, for 1 minute or until warmed through. Divide among serving bowls. Top with the extra crème fraîche, almonds and mint and coriander sprigs. Serve with the steamed rice.

## NUTRITION (PER SERVE)

| CALS | FAT | SAT FAT | PROTEIN | CARBS |
|------|-----|---------|---------|-------|
| 484 | 25g | 12g | 23g | 37g |

★★★★★

*Have made this curry so many times now. A hit with vegetarian friends.* **SRAMSEY**

○ EASY   ● FAMILY-FRIENDLY   ● GLUTEN FREE   ● LOW CAL   ● QUICK   ○ VEGAN

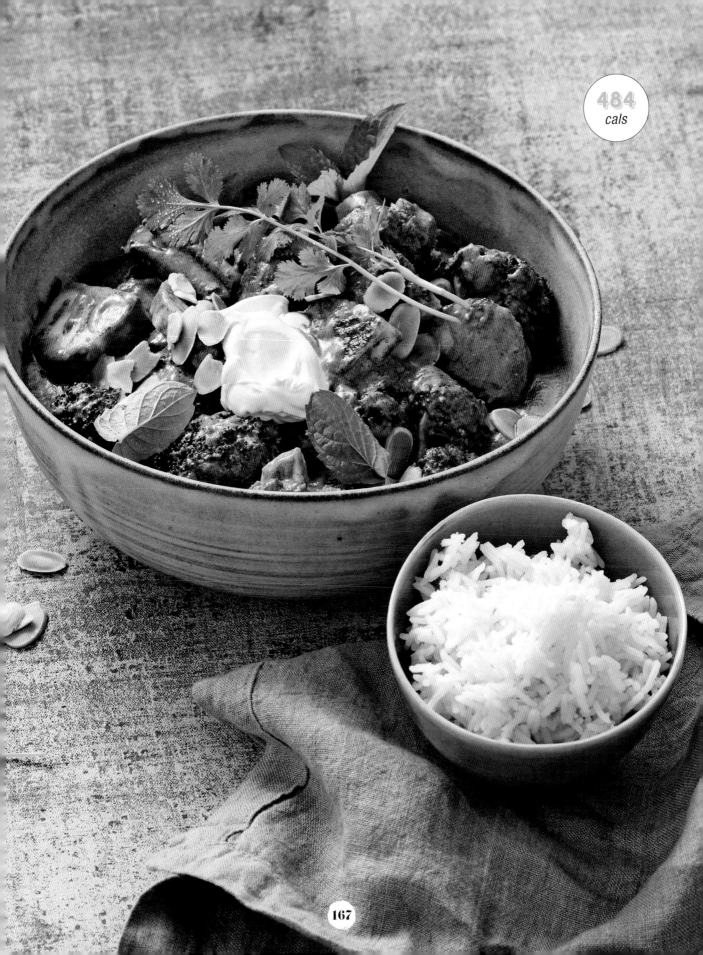

484
cals

# VEGAN STUFFED ROAST PUMPKIN

Filled with flavours like pine nuts and maple syrup, this pumpkin dish is the perfect main for vegetarians and those going totally dairy free.

**SERVES** 4  **PREP** 25 mins (+ cooling)  **COOK** 2 hours

1.8kg whole butternut pumpkin
2 red onions
1 tbs extra virgin olive oil
3 garlic cloves, thinly sliced
1 tsp smoked paprika
2 small red capsicums, deseeded, cut into 1cm-thick strips
2 small yellow capsicums, deseeded, cut into 1cm-thick strips
2 tbs red wine vinegar
2 tsp pure maple syrup
400g can brown lentils, rinsed, drained
150g baby spinach
2 tbs pine nuts
2 bunches asparagus, trimmed
Baby rocket and balsamic vinegar, to serve

1. Preheat oven to 190°C/170°C fan forced. Line a large baking tray with baking paper. Cut the pumpkin in half lengthways and scoop out the seeds. Place pumpkin halves, cut-side up, on the prepared tray. Lightly spray with oil. Season. Roast for 1 hour 10 minutes or until tender. Set aside to cool. Scoop out and reserve flesh from each pumpkin half, leaving a 3cm-thick shell.

2. Meanwhile, cut 1 onion into wedges. Thinly slice the remaining onion. Heat the oil in a large frying pan over medium heat. Cook sliced onion, stirring, for 3 minutes or until softened. Add the garlic and paprika. Cook, stirring, for 1 minute. Add the capsicum and cook, stirring occasionally, for 10 minutes or until just tender. Stir in the vinegar and maple syrup. Cook, stirring occasionally, for 10-15 minutes or until vegetables are caramelised.

3. Add the lentils and reserved pumpkin to the onion mixture. Season. Stir. Set aside to cool slightly.

4. Blanch spinach in boiling water for 30 seconds. Drain. Refresh under cold running water. Squeeze out excess liquid, then coarsely chop. Stir through the lentil mixture with the pine nuts.

5. Divide lentil mixture between pumpkin shells. Carefully join halves and use kitchen string to tie at 2cm intervals. Return pumpkin to the baking tray. Add the onion wedges. Roast for 20 minutes or until just tender, adding asparagus halfway through cooking. Set aside for 5 minutes. Serve with the asparagus, onion and rocket, and drizzled with balsamic.

## NUTRITION (PER SERVE)

| CALS | FAT | SAT FAT | PROTEIN | CARBS |
|------|-----|---------|---------|-------|
| 328 | 13.1g | 1.7g | 14.3g | 31.7g |

○ EASY   ○ FAMILY-FRIENDLY   ● GLUTEN FREE   ● LOW CAL   ○ QUICK   ● VEGAN

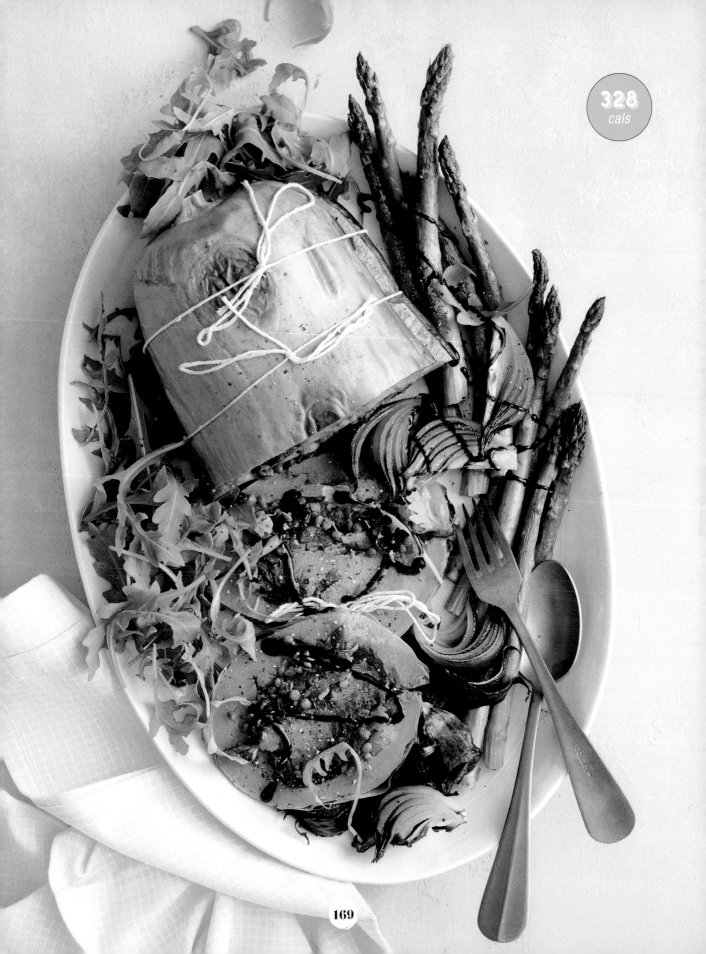

# BEAN & BEETS MUSHROOM
# BURGERS

We've swapped buns for giant mushies, and mince for mashed bean and beetroot patties, to make these ridiculously tasty gluten-free burgers.

**SERVES** 4  **PREP** 15 mins  **COOK** 15 mins

400g can red kidney beans,
  rinsed, drained
2 tsp Mexican spice seasoning
2 green shallots, finely chopped
1 egg, lightly beaten
1 small beetroot, peeled,
  coarsely grated
8 large field mushrooms,
  stalks removed
250g fresh buffalo mozzarella,
  cut into 4 slices
20g salad leaves
Sour cream, to serve
60g (⅓ cup) drained sun-dried
  tomatoes, sliced
1 avocado, sliced
Fresh coriander leaves,
  to serve

1 Place the beans in a large bowl and roughly mash. Add seasoning, shallot, egg and beetroot. Season. Stir until just combined. Divide the mixture into 4 patties.

2 Heat a large non-stick frying pan over medium heat. Spray with olive oil. Place the patties in the pan and flatten a little. Cook for 2-3 minutes each side or until golden and heated through.

3 Meanwhile, preheat an oven grill. Place mushrooms on a baking tray and spray with oil. Cook under the grill, gill-side down, for 1-2 minutes or until lightly golden. Turn over and cook for 30 seconds. Lay cheese on 4 of the mushrooms and cook for 1-2 minutes or until the cheese is golden and bubbling. Transfer to serving plates.

4 Add salad leaves to the cheese-topped mushrooms. Top with a patty, a big dollop of sour cream, sun-dried tomato, avocado and coriander. Top with the remaining mushrooms for lids and serve.

**COOK'S NOTE**

You can make the patties up to 1 day in advance. Before using, place in the microwave until heated through.

## NUTRITION (PER SERVE)

| CALS | FAT | SAT FAT | PROTEIN | CARBS |
|------|-----|---------|---------|-------|
| 520 | 37g | 18g | 23g | 17g |

● EASY  ● FAMILY-FRIENDLY  ● GLUTEN FREE  ● LOW CAL  ● QUICK  ○ VEGAN

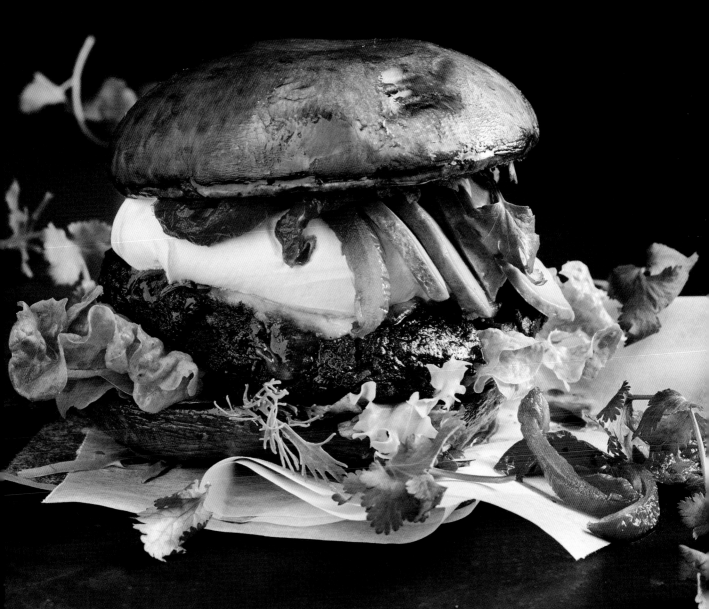

520
cals

★★★★★ *Pretty simple to make, tasty, and they actually held together which was nice. Didn't bother grilling the mushroom, just fried them and threw cheese on top — winner.* **MIK1111**

171

# 5-INGREDIENT LASAGNE

This ingenious lasagne is prepped in just 15 minutes. Each bite is a burst of cheesy, caramelised onion flavour. It's a dish the whole family will love.

**SERVES** 6 **PREP** 15 mins (+ cooling) **COOK** 30 mins

2 x 325g pkts pumpkin caramelised
  onion ravioli
400g btl tomato pasta sauce
  with basil and onion
425g tub creamy cheese sauce
155g (1½ cups) pre-grated
  4 cheese blend
60g packet baby spinach,
  coarsely chopped

1 Preheat oven to 200°C/180°C fan forced. Lightly grease a 5cm-deep 20cm square baking dish and a baking tray. Cook the ravioli in a large saucepan of salted boiling water for 3 minutes or until al dente. Drain and rinse under cold water. Drain. Transfer to the prepared tray.

2 Spread 125ml (½ cup) tomato pasta sauce over the base of the prepared dish. Top with a layer of ravioli, in rows of about 4. Dot with one-third of the cheese sauce. Smooth the surface. Sprinkle with 40g (⅓ cup) cheese and one-third of the spinach.

3 Top with another layer of ravioli. Dot with half the remaining cheese sauce. Smooth the surface. Sprinkle with half the remaining spinach and ⅓ cup cheese. Repeat with another layer of the ravioli, remaining cheese sauce, ⅓ cup cheese and remaining spinach.

4 Arrange a final layer of ravioli on top. Spread with remaining tomato pasta sauce. Sprinkle with the remaining cheese. Bake for 20-25 minutes, or until golden. Set aside for 10 minutes to cool slightly before serving.

## NUTRITION (PER SERVE)

| CALS | FAT | SAT FAT | PROTEIN | CARBS |
| --- | --- | --- | --- | --- |
| 511 | 25.7g | 16.3g | 20.2g | 47.3g |

★★★★★ *Very easy, and yum! Served ours with vegies; can't wait for leftovers tomorrow.* **JAANE93**

● EASY   ● FAMILY-FRIENDLY   ○ GLUTEN FREE   ● LOW CAL   ○ QUICK   ○ VEGAN

511
cals

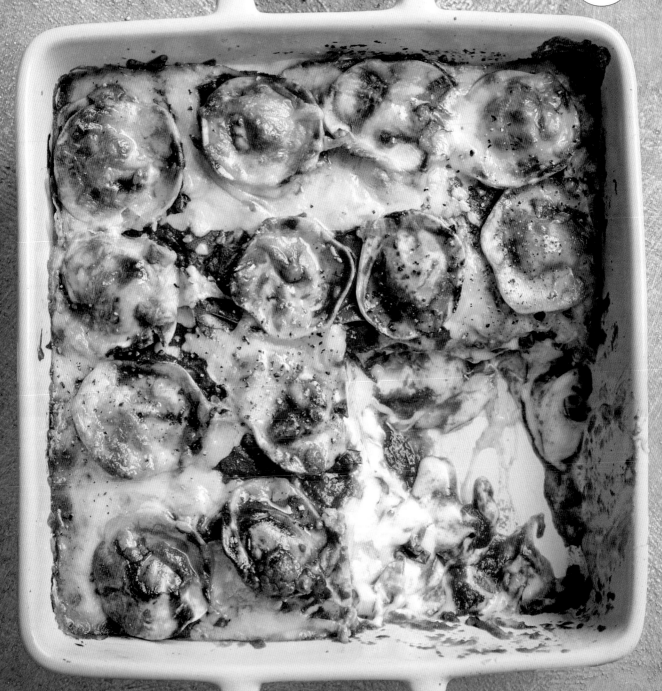

# DHAL-STUFFED SWEET POTATOES

These sweet spuds pack a health punch, thanks to the dhal, which is an excellent source of iron and fibre, and a good source of protein.

**SERVES** 6  **PREP** 15 mins  **COOK** 45 mins

6 (350g each) orange sweet potatoes
2 tbs extra virgin olive oil
1 brown onion, finely chopped
2 x 400g cans gluten-free brown lentils, rinsed, drained
2 garlic cloves, crushed
2 tsp ground cumin
2 tsp ground coriander
1 tsp garam masala
1 tsp hot paprika
2 tbs tomato paste
270ml can coconut milk
400g can diced tomatoes
1½ tbs lemon juice
Plain Greek-style yoghurt, fresh coriander sprigs and mixed salad leaves, to serve

1 Preheat oven to 200°C/180°C fan forced. Line a large baking tray with baking paper. Place potatoes on the prepared tray. Drizzle with half the oil. Season. Bake for 45 minutes or until tender. Set aside for 5 minutes to cool slightly.

2 Meanwhile, heat the remaining oil in a large frying pan over medium-high heat. Add the onion and cook, stirring, for 5 minutes or until softened. Add the lentils, garlic and spices. Cook, stirring, for 1 minute or until aromatic.

3 Add the tomato paste. Stir for 1 minute or until lentils are coated. Add the coconut milk and tomato. Bring to the boil. Reduce heat to low. Simmer, uncovered, for 10 minutes or until sauce reduces and thickens. Stir in the lemon juice. Season.

4 Cut a 1cm-thick slice from the top of each potato. Place tops in a large bowl. Holding each potato with a clean tea towel, scoop flesh from potato, leaving a 1cm shell. Transfer flesh to the bowl with the tops and coarsely mash. Fold in the lentil mixture. Spoon into potatoes. Drizzle with yoghurt and sprinkle with coriander sprigs. Serve with salad leaves.

## NUTRITION (PER SERVE)

| CALS | FAT | SAT FAT | PROTEIN | CARBS |
|------|-----|---------|---------|-------|
| 554 | 16.7g | 7.4g | 18g | 71.8g |

★★★★★

*Easy and delicious. Sooooo tasty. Definitely on repeat!* **MACOME**

● EASY  ○ FAMILY-FRIENDLY  ● GLUTEN FREE  ● LOW CAL  ○ QUICK  ○ VEGAN

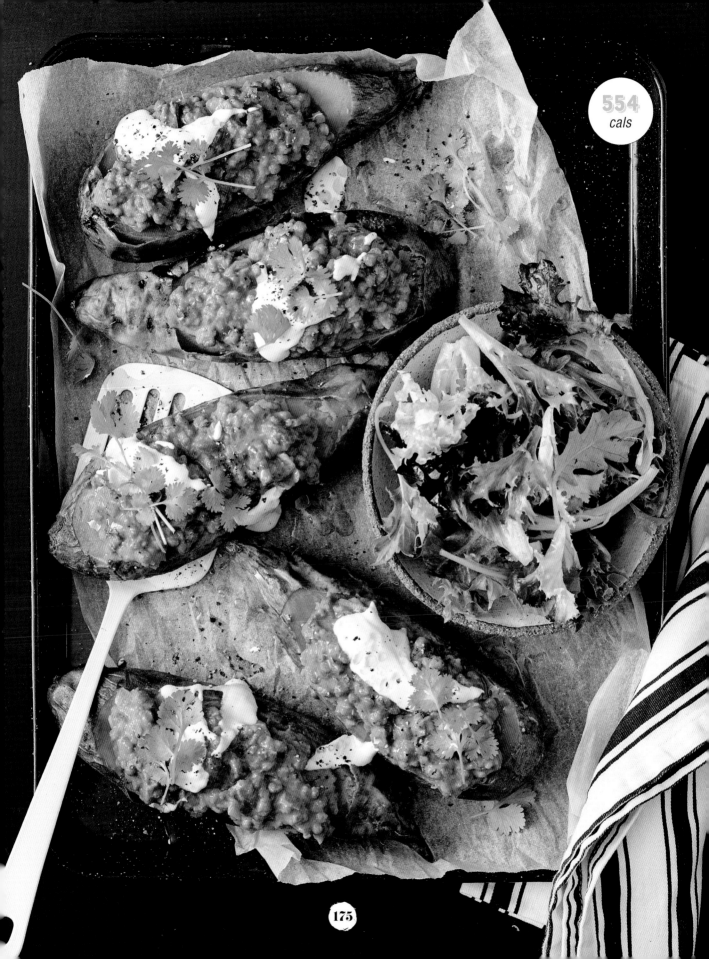

554 cals

175

# CHEESY PUMPKIN & POTATO BAKE

To make this cheesy and creamy potato bake even more filling, we added kale, pumpkins and lentils – it'll be a new family favourite after the first bite!

**MAKES** 6  **PREP** 20 mins (+ standing)  **COOK** 1 hour 25 mins

300ml pouring cream

2 tsp gluten-free vegetable stock powder

2 tbs olive oil

70g chopped kale

1 leek, halved lengthways, sliced

2 garlic cloves, crushed

½ (about 650g) butternut pumpkin, peeled, deseeded, cut into 5mm-thick slices

500g desiree potatoes, peeled, cut into 4mm-thick slices

400g can gluten-free lentils, rinsed, drained

130g (1¼ cups) pre-grated 3 cheese blend

**1** Preheat the oven to 200ºC/180ºC fan forced. Grease a 20 x 30cm baking dish. Combine the cream and stock powder in a jug and set aside.

**2** Heat 1 tbs oil in a large, deep frying pan over medium heat. Reserve a large handful of chopped kale. Add the remaining kale and 1 tbs water to the pan. Cook, stirring often, for 1-2 minutes or until the kale has wilted and the water has evaporated. Transfer to a bowl.

**3** Heat the remaining oil in the pan. Add the leek and garlic. Cook, stirring, for 2 minutes or until softened. Add to the kale. Cut each slice of pumpkin into 4-5cm pieces.

**4** Arrange a layer of sliced potato over the base of the prepared dish, overlapping slightly. Season. Top with half the kale mixture, then half the lentils. Drizzle with a little cream mixture. Top with a layer of pumpkin. Cover with the remaining kale mixture, then remaining lentils, seasoning each layer. Drizzle with a little cream mixture. Finish with a layer of the remaining potato and pumpkin. Pour over the remaining cream mixture. Cover dish with foil and bake for 1 hour.

**5** Uncover dish and top with the reserved kale. Scatter with cheese. Bake, uncovered, for 20 minutes or until golden. Stand for 10 minutes before serving.

## NUTRITION (PER SERVE)

| CALS | FAT | SAT FAT | PROTEIN | CARBS |
|------|------|---------|---------|-------|
| 451 | 32.5g | 17.9g | 14.4g | 22.9g |

○ EASY   ○ FAMILY-FRIENDLY   ● GLUTEN FREE   ● LOW CAL   ○ QUICK   ○ VEGAN

451
cals

★★★★★
*Made as per recipe. It was perfect.
My fussy three-year-old even ate it.* **SHELLEY131**

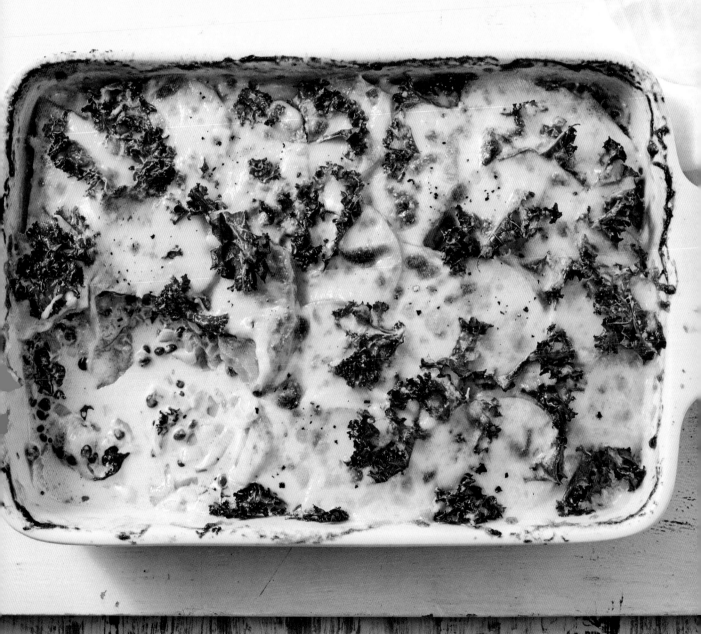

# MEXICAN BURRITO
# LASAGNE

Why have just burritos when you can have a burrito in a lasagne?!
It's a fun way to boost flavour and use up ingredients in the pantry.

**SERVES** 6  **PREP** 20 mins (+ cooling)  **COOK** 35 mins

1 tbs olive oil
1 brown onion, coarsely chopped
1 red capsicum, deseeded,
    coarsely chopped
2 garlic cloves, crushed
1 tsp Mexican chilli powder
1 tsp ground cumin
1 tsp dried oregano
300g sweet potato, peeled,
    coarsely grated
400g can diced tomatoes
400g can black beans, rinsed,
    drained
300g can corn kernels, drained
6 mini flour tortillas
155g (1½ cups) pre-grated
    Mexican cheese blend
2 green shallots, thinly sliced
2 tbs chopped fresh coriander

1. Preheat oven to 200°C/180°C fan forced. Grease a 6cm-deep, 18 x 28cm baking dish.

2. Heat the oil in a large, deep frying pan over medium heat. Add the onion and capsicum. Cook, stirring occasionally, for 5 minutes or until softened. Add the garlic, chilli powder, cumin and oregano. Cook, stirring, for 30 seconds or until aromatic. Add the sweet potato. Cook, stirring, for 3 minutes or until softened. Stir in the tomato and cook for 5 minutes or until the sweet potato is tender. Stir in the black beans and corn. Season. Set aside for 10 minutes to cool slightly.

3. Place 2 tortillas over the base of the prepared dish. Sprinkle with 35g (⅓ cup) cheese. Spread with half of the black bean mixture. Top with another 2 tortillas, ⅓ cup cheese and remaining black bean mixture. Top with the remaining 2 tortillas and sprinkle with remaining cheese.

4. Bake for 20 minutes or until golden and heated through. Sprinkle with shallot and coriander, to serve.

## NUTRITION (PER SERVE)

| CALS | FAT | SAT FAT | PROTEIN | CARBS |
| --- | --- | --- | --- | --- |
| 450 | 17.7g | 8.1g | 17.2g | 52.8g |

○ EASY  ● FAMILY-FRIENDLY  ○ GLUTEN FREE  ● LOW CAL  ○ QUICK  ○ VEGAN

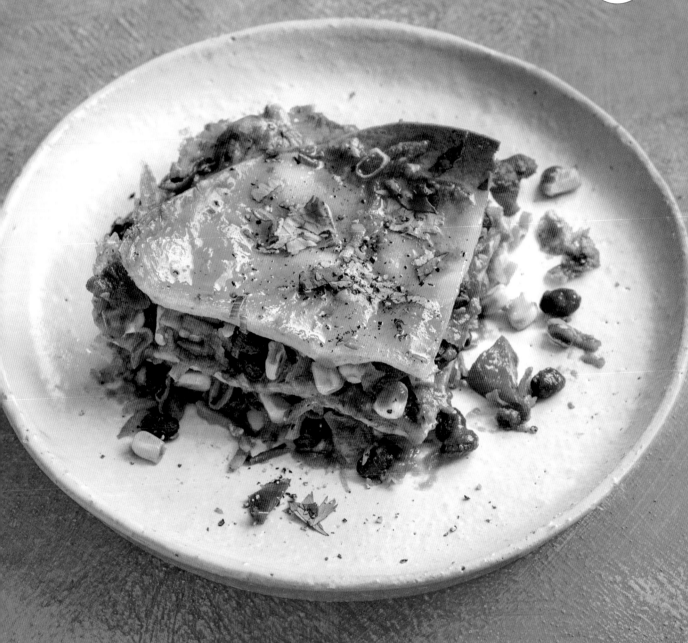

★★★★★ *Great alternative to individual burritos!*
*I didn't realise this recipe didn't have mince in it until I started*
*to cook it – it was great!* **DEBRAMCCALLUM**

# TOFU CHILLI
# ENCHILADAS

This spicy dinner explodes in tasty Mexican flavours and vegetables. The tofu adds the protein all vegetarians need for a healthier dinner.

**SERVES** 4  **PREP** 15 mins  **COOK** 30 mins

1½ tbs extra virgin olive oil
1 red onion, finely chopped
1 small red capsicum, finely chopped
1 tbs finely chopped fresh coriander leaves, root and stem
1 tbs ground cumin
2 tsp Mexican chilli powder
3 garlic cloves, crushed
2 x 410g can rich & thick diced tomatoes with paste
2 tbs water
420g can corn kernels, rinsed, drained
400g can kidney beans, rinsed, drained
300g firm tofu, cut into 1cm pieces
1 tsp balsamic vinegar
8 multigrain tortillas, warmed
40g (½ cup) reduced-fat grated cheddar
200g grape tomatoes, halved
3 green shallots, finely sliced
2 tbs chopped fresh coriander
Extra-light sour cream, to serve (optional)

**1** Preheat oven to 200°C/180°C fan forced. Lightly grease a 20 x 29cm ovenproof dish. Heat the oil in a non-stick frying pan over medium heat. Add the onion and capsicum. Cook, stirring, for 5 minutes or until softened. Add the coriander, cumin, chilli and garlic. Cook, stirring, for 2 minutes or until aromatic. Stir in 1 can tomato and the water. Simmer for 2 minutes. Add the corn, kidney beans, tofu and vinegar. Simmer, stirring, for 6 minutes or until warmed through. Season.

**2** Spread one-third of remaining tomato can over base of the prepared dish. Top 1 tortilla with one-eighth of the tofu mixture. Roll up to enclose. Place seam side down in the dish. Repeat with remaining tortillas and tofu mixture. Drizzle over remaining tomato. Sprinkle with cheese.

**3** Bake for 20 minutes or until cheese melts. Combine grape tomato, shallot and coriander in a bowl. Top enchiladas with tomato salsa and serve with sour cream, if desired.

**COOK'S NOTE**

Firm tofu is ideal for a dish like this as it retains its shape. It's also packed full of protein and absorbs the yummy chilli flavours.

## NUTRITION (PER SERVE)

| CALS | FAT | SAT FAT | PROTEIN | CARBS |
|------|-----|---------|---------|-------|
| 593 | 20g | 6g | 26.1g | 63g |

★ ★ ★ ★ ★

*Didn't have kidney beans, so diced some mushrooms instead. It was so delicious.* **JULIEJABBER**

○ EASY  ● **FAMILY-FRIENDLY**  ○ GLUTEN FREE  ● **LOW CAL**  ○ QUICK  ○ VEGAN

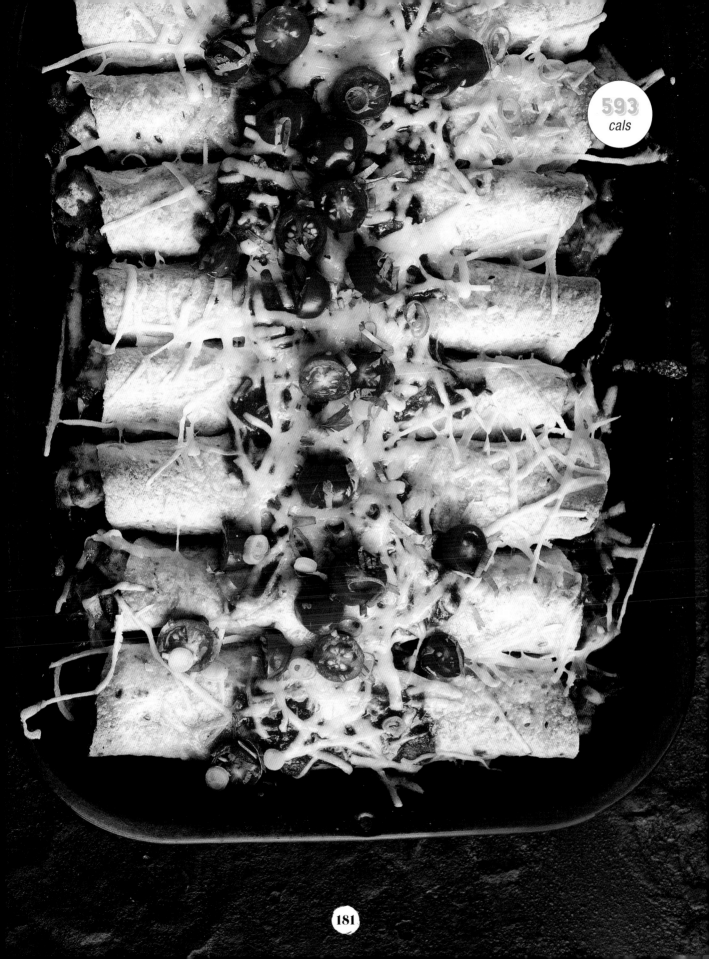

593
cals

181

# CLEAN-OUT THE FRIDGE
# RISOTTO

Get stuck into the vegie crisper for the ingredients for this veg-packed risotto. It's a great way to benefit from any leftover bits and pieces before they spoil.

**SERVES** 4-6    **PREP** 15 mins    **COOK** 35 mins

2 corncobs, husk and silk removed
1.25L (5 cups) gluten-free vegetable stock
2 tbs olive oil
1 brown onion, finely chopped
2 celery sticks, thinly sliced, leaves reserved
4 stems silverbeet, leaves torn, coarsely chopped, stalks thinly sliced
2 garlic cloves, crushed
330g (1½ cups) arborio rice
Parmesan rind, for flavour, (see note) plus finely grated parmesan, to serve
150g (1 cup) frozen peas

1. Use a sharp knife to remove the kernels from the corncobs. Set aside. Place the cobs in a saucepan. Add the stock. Cover and bring to the boil over medium heat. Reduce heat to low and leave to gently simmer.

2. Heat the oil in a large saucepan over medium heat. Add the onion, celery and silverbeet stalks. Cook, stirring often, for 5 minutes or until softened. Add the garlic and rice. Stir for 1 minute or until the grains appear slightly glassy.

3. Add 1 ladle (about 125ml/½ cup) of stock to the rice. Stir constantly with a wooden spoon until liquid is absorbed. Add half of the remaining stock, 1 ladle at a time, stirring until the liquid is absorbed before adding the next ladle, for about 10 minutes. Stir in corn kernels and parmesan rind. Add the remaining stock, 1 ladle at a time, stirring until the liquid is absorbed before adding the next ladle, for 8-10 minutes or until rice is tender yet firm to the bite and risotto is creamy.

4. Add the peas and silverbeet leaves to the rice mixture and stir until peas are heated through and silverbeet is wilted. Ladle the risotto into serving bowls. Sprinkle with the grated parmesan and reserved celery leaves, to serve.

## COOK'S NOTE

If you just have a bit of parmesan left on the rind, grate the cheese then add the rind to the pot while the rice cooks, to impart flavour. You can also add parmesan rind to minestrone or other soups for extra flavour.

## NUTRITION (PER SERVE)

| CALS | FAT | SAT FAT | PROTEIN | CARBS |
|------|-----|---------|---------|-------|
| 520 | 14g | 3.8g | 15.2g | 78.4g |

○ EASY    ● FAMILY-FRIENDLY    ● GLUTEN FREE    ● LOW CAL    ○ QUICK    ○ VEGAN

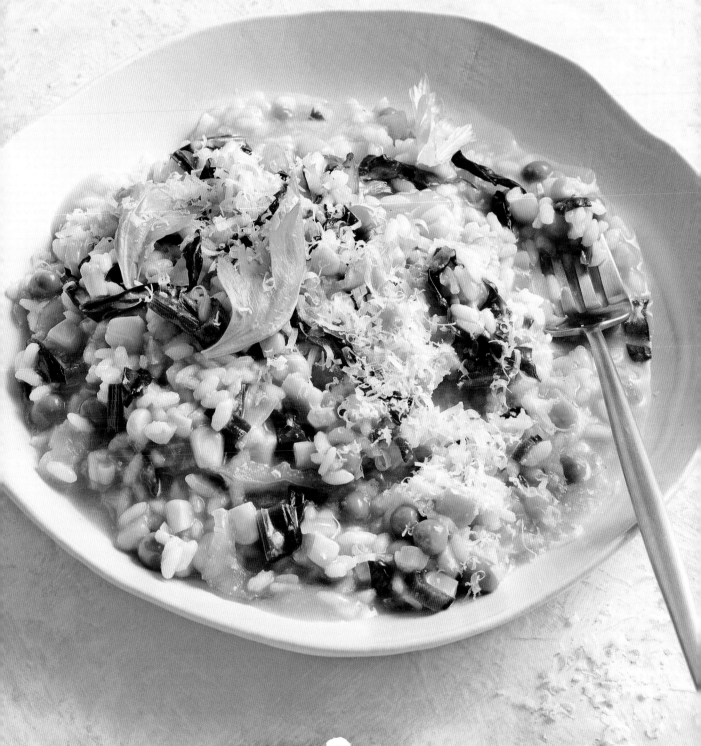

520
cals

# CAULIFLOWER PARMIGIANA
# TRAY BAKE

Cauliflower makes for a low-cal, high-fibre version of the pub 'parmy'. Smothered in a veg-laden sauce, it's a more nutritious choice, too.

**SERVES** 4  **PREP** 15 mins  **COOK** 50 mins

1 head cauliflower
1 tsp dried oregano leaves
1 small (about 400g) eggplant, cut into 1cm-thick rounds
1 tbs extra virgin olive oil
1 small red onion, finely chopped
1 small carrot, finely chopped
3 garlic cloves, thinly sliced
2 truss tomatoes, finely chopped
400g can diced tomatoes
1 tsp balsamic vinegar
60ml (¼ cup) water
¼ cup fresh basil, torn, plus extra, to serve
90g bocconcini, drained, sliced
Baby spinach, to serve

1 Preheat the oven to 200°C/180°C fan forced. Line a large baking tray with baking paper. Cut cauliflower into 1.5m-thick slices (depending on the size of your cauliflower, you will get 4-6 slices). Place slices on the prepared tray and lightly spray with oil. Season. Sprinkle with oregano. Bake for 10 minutes. Arrange eggplant around the cauliflower and spray with oil. Bake, turning once during cooking, for 30 minutes or until vegies are golden and tender.

2 Meanwhile, heat the oil in a saucepan over medium heat. Add the onion and carrot. Cook, stirring, for 5 minutes or until softened. Add the garlic and truss tomato. Cook, stirring, for 2-3 minutes or until softened. Add the diced tomato, vinegar and water. Simmer gently for 10 minutes or until the sauce is thickened. Stir through the basil.

3 Place eggplant slices on top of the cauliflower. Spoon the tomato mixture over the top. Arrange bocconcini on each stack and bake for 5-10 minutes or until the cheese is melted and golden. Serve with baby spinach.

## NUTRITION (PER SERVE)

| CALS | FAT | SAT FAT | PROTEIN | CARBS |
|------|-----|---------|---------|-------|
| 234 | 12.8g | 4.4g | 10.9g | 15.4g |

● EASY  ○ FAMILY-FRIENDLY  ● GLUTEN FREE  ● LOW CAL  ○ QUICK  ○ VEGAN

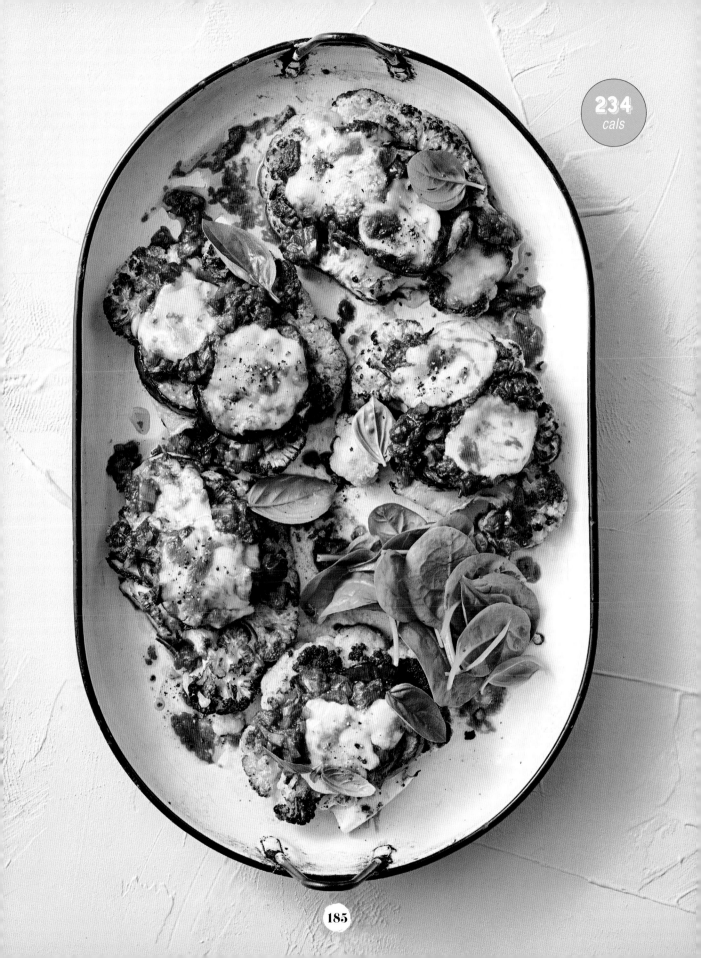

# BLACK BEAN & CHIPOTLE SOUP

With four serves of veg per person, our Mexican-inspired soup is jam-packed with antioxidants. It's also gluten-free, and low in fat and calories. Olé!

**SERVES** 4  **PREP** 20 mins  **COOK** 30 mins

1 tbs extra virgin olive oil
1 large brown onion, finely chopped
2 celery sticks, finely chopped
2 carrots, peeled, finely chopped
2 garlic cloves, crushed
2 tsp smoked paprika
2 tsp ground cumin
1 tbs chipotle in adobo sauce
3 truss tomatoes, finely chopped
70g (⅓ cup) quinoa, rinsed, drained
400g can black beans, rinsed, drained
500ml (2 cups) gluten-free vegetable stock
500ml (2 cups) water
1 large zucchini, thinly sliced
150g (1 cup) fresh corn kernels
1 tbs fresh lime juice, plus lime wedges, to serve
¼ cup chopped fresh coriander leaves, plus extra sprigs, to serve

**1** Heat the oil in a large saucepan over medium heat. Cook the onion, celery and carrot, stirring, for 5 minutes or until softened. Add the garlic, paprika, cumin and chipotle. Cook, stirring, for 1 minute or until aromatic. Add the tomato and cook, stirring occasionally, for 2-3 minutes or until starting to break down. Add the quinoa, black beans, stock and water. Bring to the boil. Reduce heat to low. Simmer, partially covered, for 15 minutes or until the quinoa is tender.

**2** Add the zucchini and corn to the pan. Simmer for 5 minutes or until vegetables are tender. Stir in the lime juice and coriander. Season. Top with extra coriander sprigs. Serve with extra lime wedges.

## COOK'S NOTE

Chipotle is dried, smoked jalapeño chillies, usually combined with a spicy adobo sauce. You'll find it in cans or jars in the Mexican food section of the supermarket.

## NUTRITION (PER SERVE)

| CALS | FAT | SAT FAT | PROTEIN | CARBS |
|------|-----|---------|---------|-------|
| 304 | 7.5g | 1g | 13g | 39g |

○ EASY    ○ FAMILY-FRIENDLY    ● GLUTEN FREE    ● LOW CAL    ○ QUICK    ○ VEGAN

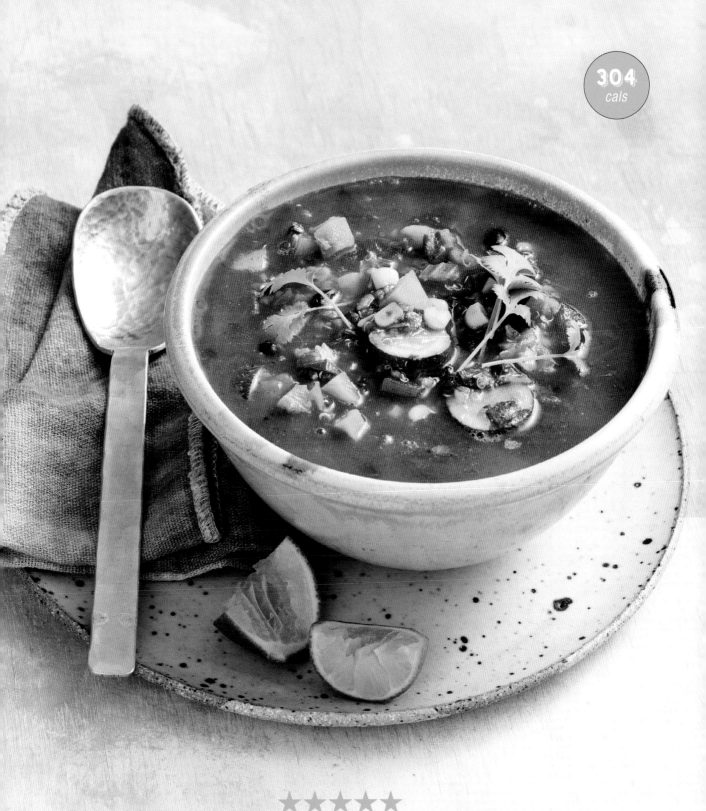

★★★★★

*Very warming and super-filling soup.* JNNPYRZ

304 cals

187

# SMOKY EGGPLANT & BEAN
# STEW

This low-cal dish is HUGE on flavour. We've added red kidney beans, which are low GI and high in protein, kicking up the healthy factor a notch or two.

**SERVES** 4  **PREP** 20 mins  **COOK** 45 mins

1 tbs extra virgin olive oil

2 small or 1 large eggplant, cut into 2cm pieces

1 large red onion, finely chopped

3 celery sticks, cut into 1cm pieces

2 garlic cloves, thinly sliced

2-3 tsp harissa paste, to taste

1 tsp smoked paprika, plus extra, to serve

1 tsp ground cumin

400g can red kidney beans, rinsed, drained

400g can diced tomatoes

125ml (½ cup) water

300g (2 cups) cooked quinoa

Steamed broccolini, to serve

90g (⅓ cup) coconut yoghurt

1 Preheat oven to 170°C/150°C fan forced. Heat half the oil in a large flameproof casserole dish over high heat. Cook the eggplant, in 2 batches, stirring, for 3-4 minutes or until browned. Transfer to a plate.

2 Heat the remaining oil in the dish over medium heat. Add the onion and celery. Cook, stirring often, for 5 minutes or until softened. Add the garlic, harissa, paprika and cumin. Cook, stirring, for 1 minute or until aromatic. Add the kidney beans, tomato, eggplant and water. Stir to combine. Bring to the boil.

3 Cover dish and bake for 30 minutes or until the eggplant is very tender. Divide the quinoa and stew among serving plates. Serve with broccolini, a dollop of yoghurt and a sprinkle of extra paprika.

## COOK'S NOTE

This will keep well for a couple of days in the fridge – in fact, the flavour will improve as it mellows. Simply reheat in the microwave for an easy meal.

## NUTRITION (PER SERVE)

| CALS | FAT | SAT FAT | PROTEIN | CARBS |
|------|------|---------|---------|-------|
| 307 | 10.6g | 4.1g | 12.1g | 33.4g |

○ EASY  ○ FAMILY-FRIENDLY  ● GLUTEN FREE  ● LOW CAL  ○ QUICK  ● VEGAN

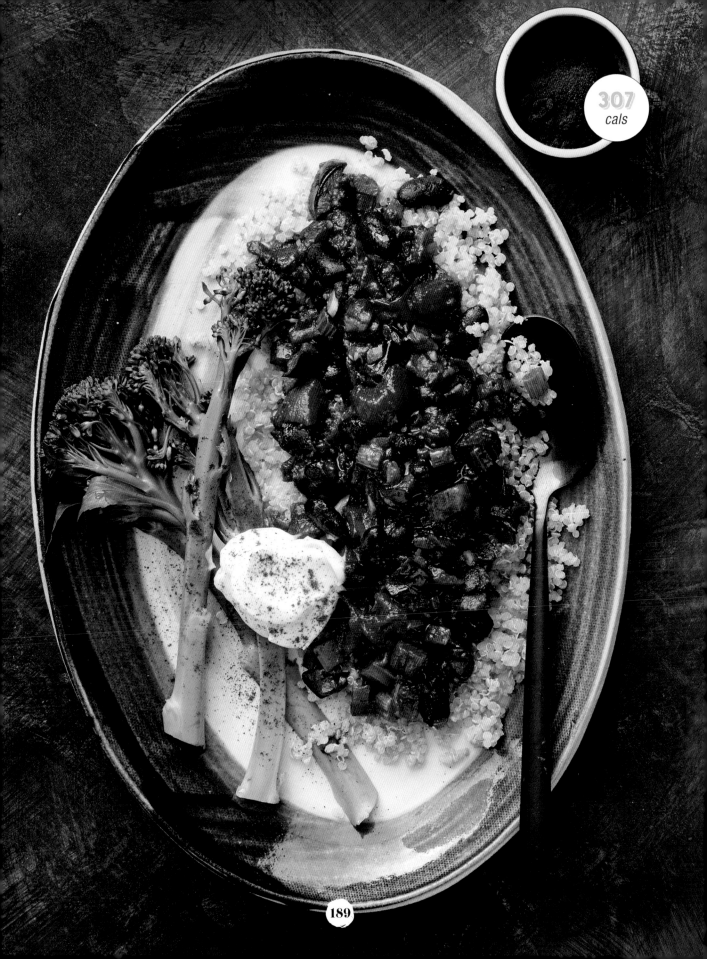

307
cals

189

# VEGAN SWEET POTATO PIE

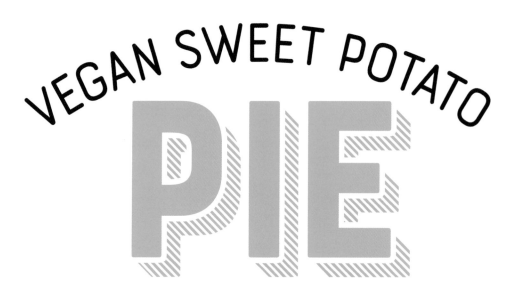

This protein-packed pie is lighter on the calories and vegan to boot, so you can keep your health kick going while enjoying the comfort foods you love.

**SERVES** 4  **PREP** 20 mins  **COOK** 1 hour 35 mins

1 tbs extra virgin olive oil
1 red onion, finely chopped
1 large carrot, finely chopped
3 celery sticks, finely chopped
2 garlic cloves, crushed
2 tsp sweet paprika
1 tsp dried oregano leaves
2 tbs no-added-salt tomato paste
400g can four bean mix, rinsed,
    drained
400g can diced tomatoes
400g can lentils, rinsed, drained
2 tsp balsamic vinegar
185ml (¾ cup) water
60g baby spinach
250g sweet potato, peeled,
    thinly sliced (see note)
250g Carisma potatoes (or other
    low-GI variety), peeled,
    thinly sliced (see note)
2 tsp fresh thyme leaves, plus thyme
    sprigs, to serve

1 Preheat the oven to 190°C/170°C fan forced. Heat the oil in a 1L (4 cup) flameproof roasting pan over medium heat. Add the onion, carrot and celery. Cook, stirring, for 5-6 minutes or until softened. Add the garlic, paprika and oregano. Cook, stirring, for 1-2 minutes or until aromatic. Add the tomato paste and cook, stirring, for 1 minute. Add the beans, tomato, lentils, balsamic vinegar and water. Bring to the boil. Reduce heat to low. Simmer for 10-15 minutes or until the sauce has thickened. Season.

2 Top the lentil mixture with the spinach. Arrange the sweet potato and potato over the top, overlapping slightly. Spray with oil. Sprinkle with thyme.

3 Cover the dish with foil and bake for 20 minutes. Remove the foil and bake for a further 50 minutes or until the potatoes are tender and golden. Scatter pie with the thyme sprigs, to serve.

## COOK'S NOTE

Beautifully thin and uniform potato slices can be achieved using a mandoline.

## NUTRITION (PER SERVE)

| CALS | FAT | SAT FAT | PROTEIN | CARBS |
|------|------|---------|---------|-------|
| 318 | 7.6g | 1.2g | 14.1g | 42g |

○ EASY  ○ FAMILY-FRIENDLY  ● **GLUTEN FREE**  ● **LOW CAL**  ○ QUICK  ● **VEGAN**

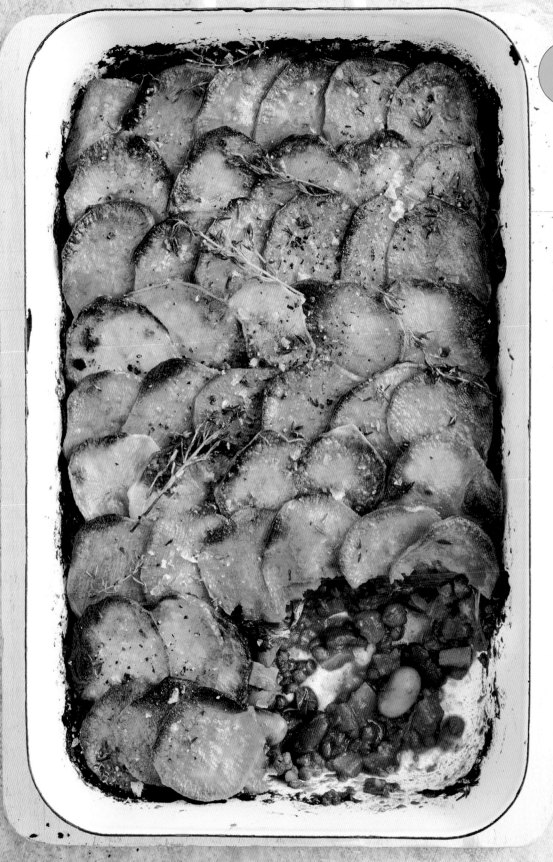

76
cals

# PUMPKIN & KALE LAZY LASAGNE

This quick and easy lasagne can be on the dinner table in just 30 minutes. There's no fiddly fitting of the pasta sheets – just stack and serve!

**SERVES** 4  **PREP** 15 mins  **COOK** 15 mins

1.5 x 375g pkt (12 small sheets) fresh lasagne
600g butternut pumpkin, peeled, deseeded, cut into 1cm pieces
2½ tbs extra virgin olive oil, plus extra, to serve
2 tbs pepitas
1½ tsp ground coriander
2 large French shallots, finely chopped
1 long fresh red chilli, thinly sliced
2 garlic cloves, crushed
1½ tsp brown mustard seeds
2 x 140g pkt chopped fresh kale
1½ tbs fresh lemon juice
250g tub cottage cheese

1 Line 2 baking trays with clean tea towels. Cook the lasagne, in batches, in a large saucepan of salted boiling water for 3-4 minutes or until al dente. Transfer pasta to the prepared trays to drain.

2 Meanwhile, place the pumpkin in a microwave-safe bowl. Microwave, covered, for 2 minutes or until starting to soften. Drain.

3 Heat 1 tbs oil in a frying pan over medium-high heat. Cook the pumpkin, stirring, for 5 minutes or until tender. Add pepitas and coriander. Season. Cook, stirring, for 1 minute or until aromatic. Transfer to a bowl.

4 Heat remaining oil in the pan over medium heat. Add the French shallot. Cook, stirring, for 2 minutes or until softened. Add chilli, garlic and mustard. Stir for 1 minute or until aromatic. Add kale. Cook, stirring, for 4 minutes or until just tender. Stir in lemon juice. Cook for 1 minute. Season.

5 Place a sheet of lasagne on each serving plate. Top with a spoonful of cottage cheese and one-third of the pumpkin mixture. Spoon over one-third of the kale mixture. Repeat layering, finishing with the kale mixture. Drizzle with extra oil. Season with black pepper and serve.

## COOK'S NOTE

You can replace the kale with any leafy greens you have on hand – try subbing in English or baby spinach, silverbeet or rainbow chard.

## NUTRITION (PER SERVE)

| CALS | FAT | SAT FAT | PROTEIN | CARBS |
| --- | --- | --- | --- | --- |
| 136 | 24g | 5g | 24g | 58g |

● EASY  ○ FAMILY-FRIENDLY  ○ GLUTEN FREE  ● LOW CAL  ● QUICK  ○ VEGAN

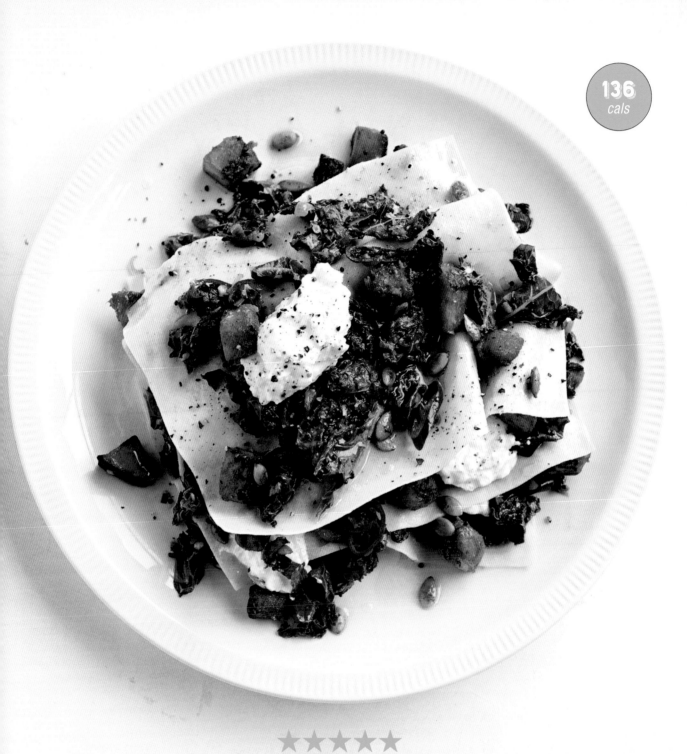

★★★★★

*I was worried it would be a little too spicy whilst cooking the kale, but when everything came together, the flavours blended well. Neither myself or my husband are vegetarian, but will definitely make again. We both loved it.* **ADMIN.FORSTER**

# CURRIED LENTIL & VEGETABLE PIE

For a hearty meal, this flavoursome lentil and veg pie hits the spot.
The slosh of curry paste will help warm you from your toes to your nose.

**SERVES** 6  **PREP** 20 mins  **COOK** 50 mins

800g cream delight potatoes, peeled
60g butter, chopped
2 tbs extra virgin olive oil
1 medium brown onion,
    finely chopped
2 garlic cloves, crushed
4cm-piece fresh ginger, finely grated
1 celery stalk, finely chopped
1 carrot, finely chopped
60g (¼ cup) Madras curry paste
2 x 400g cans gluten-free lentils,
    rinsed, drained
400g can crushed tomatoes
165ml can coconut milk
150g (1 cup) frozen peas
2 tbs fresh coriander leaves,
    to serve

**1** Place the potatoes in a large saucepan. Cover with cold water. Bring to the boil over medium-high heat and cook for 20 minutes or until tender. Drain. Transfer to a bowl and mash. Add butter and season. Stir to combine.

**2** Meanwhile, preheat oven to 220°C/200°C fan forced. Heat the oil in a large saucepan over medium heat. Add the onion, garlic, ginger, celery and carrot. Cook, stirring, for 10 minutes or until the vegetables soften.

**3** Add the curry paste. Cook, stirring, for 1 minute or until aromatic. Add the lentils, tomato and coconut milk. Bring to the boil. Reduce heat to medium-low and simmer, uncovered, for 10 minutes or until thickened. Stir in the peas.

**4** Grease a 6cm-deep, 19cm x 26cm (8-cup) oval baking dish. Spoon lentil mixture into the prepared dish. Top with mashed potato, spreading to cover. Bake for 25 minutes or until light golden. Serve topped with coriander.

## COOK'S NOTE

To make ahead, prepare the mash and curry to the end of step 3. Cool. Spoon into separate airtight containers and keep in the fridge for up to 2 days. Use a potato masher to soften the mash before using. Continue with step 4, to serve.

## NUTRITION (PER SERVE)

| CALS | FAT | SAT FAT | PROTEIN | CARBS |
|------|-----|---------|---------|-------|
| 403 | 24.7g | 10.7g | 10.8g | 30.8g |

○ EASY  ● FAMILY-FRIENDLY  ● GLUTEN FREE  ● LOW CAL  ○ QUICK  ○ VEGAN

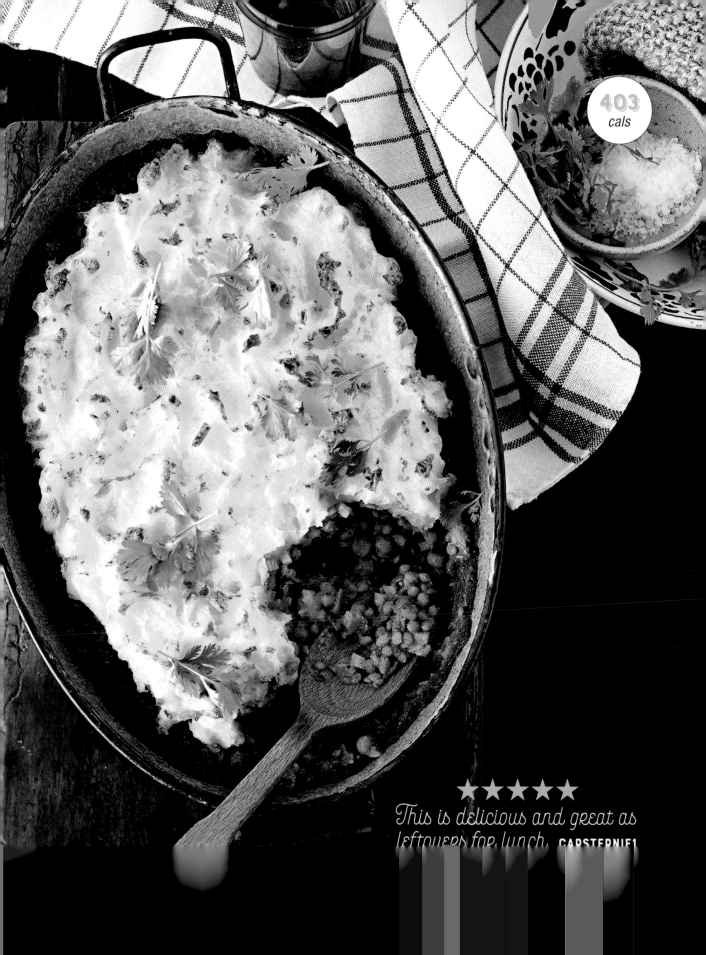

403
cals

★★★★★
This is delicious and great as
leftovers for lunch. CARSTERNIE1

# SUPER VEG ZUCCHINI CANNELLONI

We've ditched the pasta for ribbons of zucchini to wrap our yummo filling of folate-rich leafy greens and low-fat ricotta. This recipe will be on high rotation.

**SERVES** 4  **PREP** 30 mins  **COOK** 35 mins

500g jar gluten-free red wine and garlic pasta sauce
½ x 150g pkt broccoli, spinach and beet leaves
4 large zucchini, trimmed
450g fresh ricotta
1 egg yolk
1 garlic clove, crushed
1 tsp finely grated lemon rind
¼ cup finely shredded fresh basil leaves, plus extra leaves, to serve
30g (¼ cup) pre-grated mozzarella
2 tbs finely grated parmesan
Mixed salad leaves, to serve

**1** Preheat oven to 200°C/180°C fan forced. Grease a 4cm-deep, 20cm x 23cm (base) metal baking dish.

**2** Spread the pasta sauce evenly over the base of the prepared dish. Place the salad leaves in a microwave-safe bowl. Cover. Microwave for 1 minute 30 seconds or until leaves are wilted. Cool for 5 minutes. Coarsely chop.

**3** Meanwhile, using a vegetable peeler, cut 1 side of zucchini from top to bottom into long ribbons until you reach the core. Turn zucchini over. Continue cutting zucchini into ribbons until about 1cm of core is left. (Use core and small outer ribbons for another dish.) Repeat with remaining zucchini.

**4** Place ricotta, egg yolk, garlic, lemon rind, basil and chopped leaves in a bowl. Season and stir well to combine. To make each cannelloni, place 4 wide zucchini ribbons on a work surface slightly overlapping. Place 2 tbs ricotta mixture along 1 short end and roll up to enclose filling. Place, seam-side down, over sauce in dish. You will have 12 in total.

**5** Sprinkle cannelloni with mozzarella and parmesan. Spray with olive oil. Bake for 25-30 minutes or until golden. Sprinkle with extra basil leaves and serve with salad leaves.

## NUTRITION (PER SERVE)

| CALS | FAT | SAT FAT | PROTEIN | CARBS |
|------|------|---------|---------|-------|
| 313 | 16.6g | 10.1g | 17.9g | 18.5g |

○ EASY   ● FAMILY-FRIENDLY   ● GLUTEN FREE   ● LOW CAL   ○ QUICK   ○ VEGAN

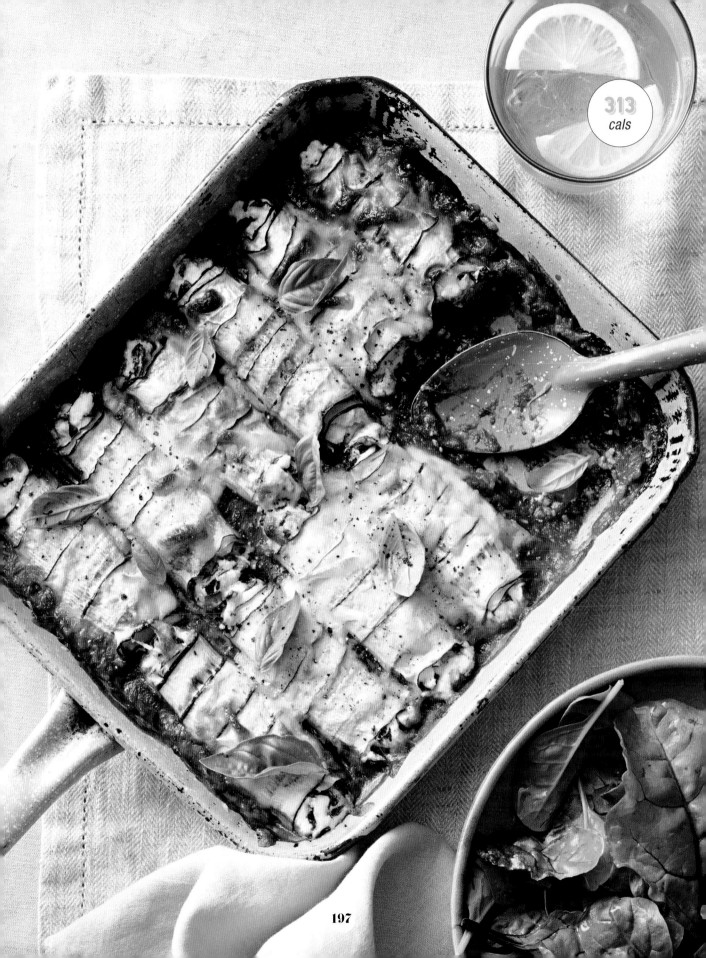

313
cals

# MEXICAN MUSHROOM TACOS

Looking to change up Taco Tuesdays? Serve up these Mexican mushroom tacos with lime-spiked avocado and the whole family will enjoy the fiesta!

**SERVES** 4  **PREP** 10 mins  **COOK** 15 mins

375g portobello mushrooms, halved
1 tsp smoked paprika
1 tsp ground cumin
1 tsp ground coriander
1 tsp dried oregano leaves
1½ tbs olive oil
1 corncob, husk and silk removed
350g pkt kaleslaw with herb yoghurt dressing
1 large avocado
2 tbs fresh lime juice
10 mini flour tortillas
1 long fresh green chilli, thinly sliced
50g feta, crumbled
Green shallots, cut lengthways into thin strips, to serve

1 Place the mushroom in a large bowl. Add paprika, cumin, coriander, oregano and oil. Toss to coat. Heat a barbecue grill or chargrill pan to medium-high. Cook the spice- and herb-coated mushroom and corn, turning, for 10 minutes or until lightly charred and tender. Transfer mushroom to a plate and the corn to a chopping board.

2 Meanwhile, place kaleslaw and dressing in a bowl. Season. Toss gently to combine. Place avocado and lime juice in a small bowl. Season. Use back of a fork to mash until mostly smooth.

3 Add tortillas to the grill, in batches, and cook, turning, for 1-2 minutes or until charred and warmed through.

4 Use a sharp knife to cut down the length of the corncob to remove the kernels. Discard cob. Spread avocado on tortillas. Top with kaleslaw, chilli, mushroom, corn, feta and shallot. Serve immediately.

**COOK'S NOTE**

Use it up! Feta is so versatile. Slice it and bake with lemon, herbs and garlic for a cheese board or snack.

## NUTRITION (PER SERVE)

| CALS | FAT | SAT FAT | PROTEIN | CARBS |
|------|------|---------|---------|-------|
| 585 | 36.6g | 8.4g | 13.9g | 43.8g |

○ EASY  ● FAMILY-FRIENDLY  ○ GLUTEN FREE  ● LOW CAL  ● QUICK  ○ VEGAN

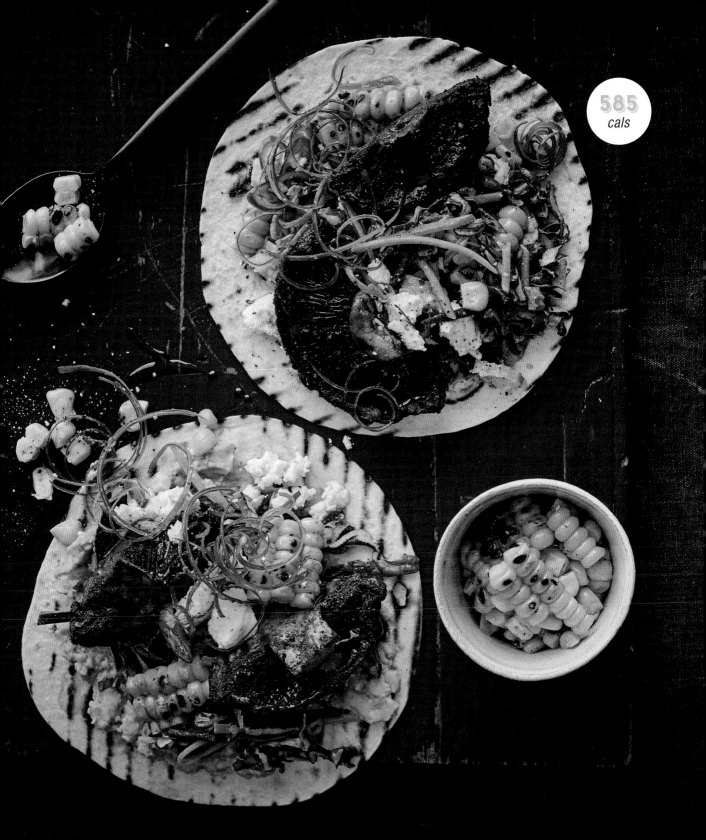

585
*cals*

★★★★★ *Loved by all. Will definitely be cooking again.* BREEBEE25

# CAPRESE LASAGNE ROLL-UPS

This family favourite mash-up turns lasagne into cannelloni with only 10 minutes prep and a handful of ingredients. You'll really want to try this one.

**SERVES** 4  **PREP** 10 mins  **COOK** 45 mins

500g fresh ricotta
125g pkt semi-dried tomato strips
½ cup chopped fresh basil leaves, plus extra leaves, to serve
150g (1½ cups) pre-grated mozzarella
4 fresh lasagne sheets
400g btl tomato basil pasta sauce
60ml (¼ cup) water

1 Preheat oven to 180°C/160°C fan forced. Grease a 1.5L (6 cup) ovenproof dish with olive oil. Place the ricotta, semi-dried tomato, basil and 1 cup mozzarella in a large bowl. Season well. Use a wooden spoon to stir until well combined.

2 Spoon a heaped ½ cup of the filling along 1 long edge of each lasagne sheet. Roll up firmly to enclose. Use a sharp knife to cut each log into 8 pieces.

3 Combine pasta sauce and water in a jug and pour two-thirds into the prepared dish. Arrange roll-ups, cut side up, over the top. Spoon over remaining sauce mixture. Sprinkle with remaining cheese. Bake for 45 minutes or until golden and tender. Top with extra basil leaves, to serve.

**COOK'S NOTE**

For a protein boost, add a 400g can brown lentils, rinsed and drained, to the ricotta mixture.

## NUTRITION (PER SERVE)

| CALS | FAT | SAT FAT | PROTEIN | CARBS |
|------|-----|---------|---------|-------|
| 591 | 33.6g | 16.3g | 28.2g | 41.5g |

★★★★★ *This looks much harder than it was to make. I made two and froze one for another dinner.* **MURRAYMINT**

● EASY  ● FAMILY-FRIENDLY  ○ GLUTEN FREE  ● LOW CAL  ○ QUICK  ○ VEGAN

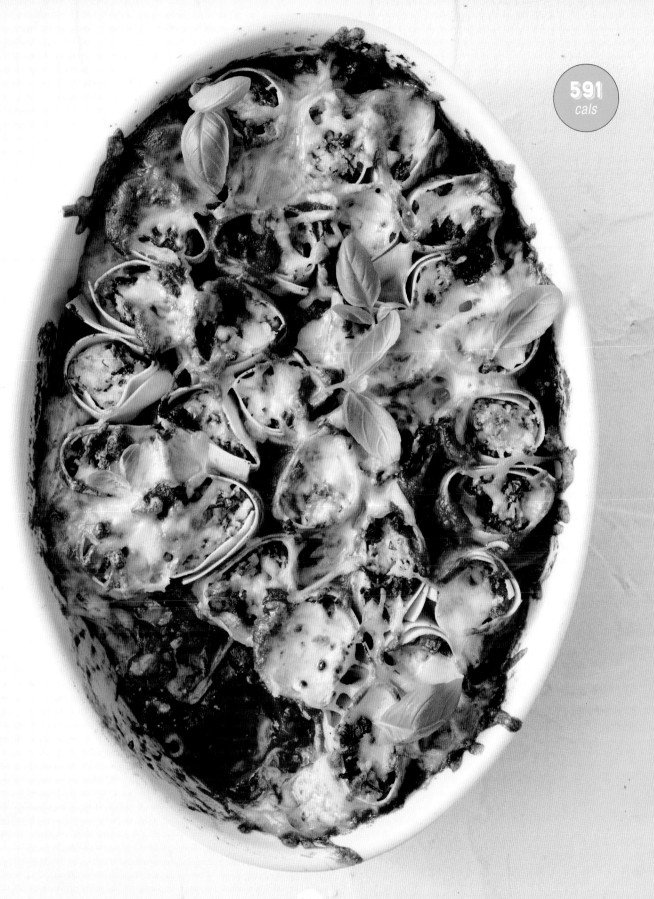

# STICKY SWEET CHILLI EGG
# NASI GORENG

A popular Indonesian stir-fry, the whole family will love these bowls of vibrant vegie goodness. The egg on top is the crowning glory.

**SERVES** 4   **PREP** 15 mins   **COOK** 15 mins

270g (1⅓ cups) long grain white rice (see note)
2 tbs vegetable oil
150g green beans, trimmed, cut into 3cm lengths
4 green shallots, thinly sliced,
50g (1 cup) frozen peas, corn and capsicum mix
1½ tbs kecap manis
4 eggs
105g (⅓ cup) sweet chilli sauce
1½ tbs lime juice
Sliced tomato and baby cucumber, sliced lengthways, to serve
1 long red chilli, thinly sliced
1 tbs fried shallots
¼ cup fresh coriander leaves
Lime wedges, to serve

1 Cook the rice following packet directions. Meanwhile, heat a wok over high heat. Add half the oil and swirl to coat. Add beans. Cook, stirring occasionally, for 3 minutes or until lightly charred. Add shallot and cook, stirring, for 1 minute. Add rice and vegie mix. Cook, stirring, for 1 minute. Add kecap manis and cook, stirring, for 2 minutes or until hot.

2 Meanwhile, heat remaining oil in a frying pan over medium-high heat. Break 2 eggs into the pan. Cook for 2 minutes or until whites are set but yolks are still runny. Turn eggs over. Cook for 20 seconds. Transfer to a plate and cover to keep warm. Repeat with remaining eggs.

3 Place the sweet chilli sauce and lime juice in a small saucepan. Heat over medium heat for 2 minutes or until simmering.

4 Divide rice mixture among 4 serving bowls. Top each with an egg, tomato and cucumber. Drizzle with chilli sauce mixture. Sprinkle with chilli, fried shallots and coriander leaves. Serve with lime wedges.

**COOK'S NOTE**

You can use leftover cooked rice for this dish and skip step 1. You'll need 4 cups cooked rice, or a 450g packet of microwave long grain white rice, heated.

## NUTRITION (PER SERVE)

| CALS | FAT | SAT FAT | PROTEIN | CARBS |
|------|-----|---------|---------|-------|
| 566 | 14.9g | 2.6g | 15.5g | 87.3g |

○ EASY   ● FAMILY-FRIENDLY   ○ GLUTEN FREE   ● LOW CAL   ● QUICK   ○ VEGAN

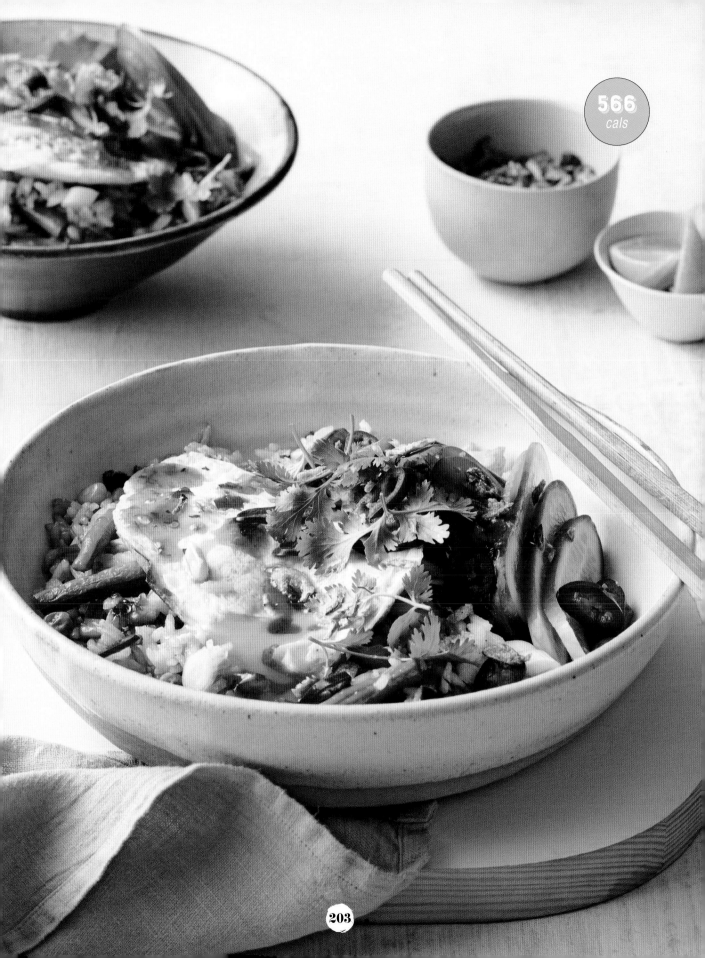

566
cals

203

# EASY FALAFEL TRAY BAKE

Masses of flavour collide in this colourful one-tray meal. With only 10 minutes prep, this is a fuss-free midweek dinner everyone will love.

**SERVES** 4  **PREP** 10 mins  **COOK** 45 mins

1 bunch baby carrots, trimmed, halved
1 red onion, cut into wedges
1 each of red and yellow capsicums, deseeded, thickly sliced
2 tbs extra virgin olive oil
200g baby truss tomatoes
1 tbs dukkah
390g pkt gluten-free falafel
½ cup fresh mint leaves

**TAHINI YOGHURT**
90g (⅓ cup) Greek-style yoghurt
3 tsp fresh lemon juice
2 tsp hulled tahini

1. Preheat oven to 210°C/190°C fan forced. Line a large baking tray with baking paper. Place carrots, onion and capsicum on the prepared tray. Drizzle with oil. Season. Roast for 20 minutes. Add the tomatoes. Roast for 15 minutes or until vegetables are golden and tender.
2. Meanwhile, to make the tahini yoghurt, combine the yoghurt, lemon juice and tahini in a small bowl. Season.
3. Sprinkle vegetables with dukkah and top with falafel. Roast for 8-10 minutes or until warmed through. Sprinkle with mint leaves and serve with tahini yoghurt.

## NUTRITION (PER SERVE)

| CALS | FAT | SAT FAT | PROTEIN | CARBS |
| --- | --- | --- | --- | --- |
| 444 | 30.8g | 4.2g | 11g | 25.8g |

**COOK'S NOTE**

For a vegan option, replace the Greek yoghurt with plain coconut yoghurt and increase the tahini to 3 tsp. Also check your chosen falafel is vegan.

★★★★★

*The falafel, dukkah, and yoghurt sauce on this easy vegie tray bake made it a real winner in our family — even the non-vegetarians loved it.*

**CHARLIEDINNERS**

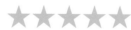

● EASY  ● FAMILY-FRIENDLY  ● GLUTEN FREE  ● LOW CAL  ○ QUICK  ○ VEGAN

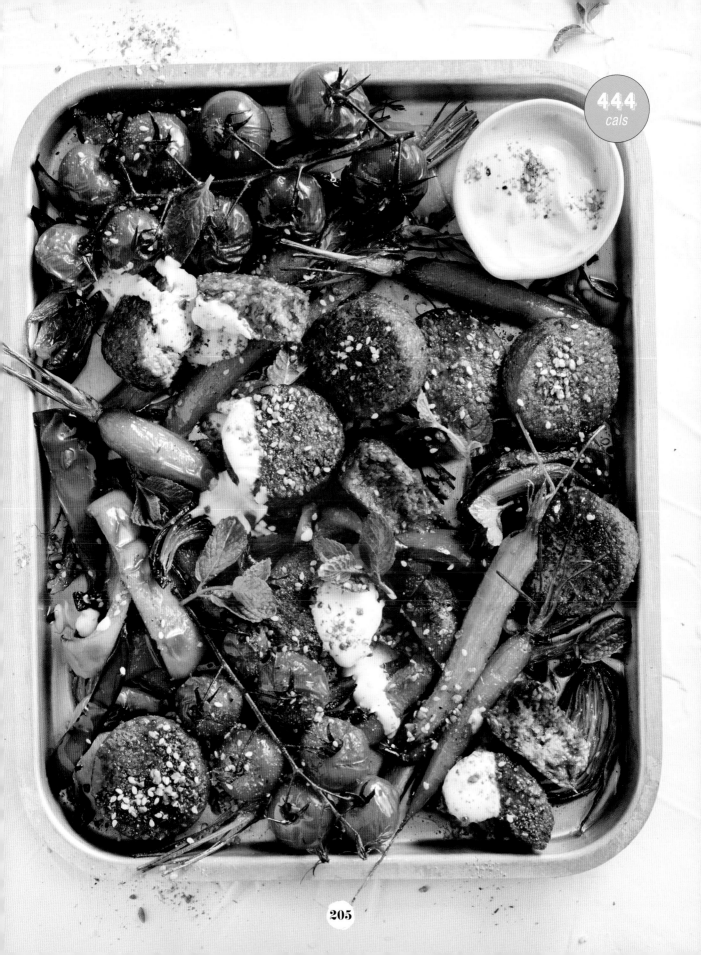

444
cals

205

# SPRING VEGETABLES &

# HALOUMI

Plate up this good-for-you satisfying main. Abundant in vibrant vegies, protein, vitamin C and magnesium, it's a great way to end any day.

**SERVES** 4  **PREP** 20 mins (+ cooling)  **COOK** 30 mins

200g (1 cup) brown rice
1 bunch baby carrots, trimmed, peeled
1 bunch broccolini, trimmed
1 bunch asparagus, trimmed
60ml (¼ cup) extra virgin olive oil, plus extra 2 tsp
2 tbs fresh lemon juice, plus shredded lemon rind and lemon halves, to serve
1 tsp honey
250g haloumi, thinly sliced
¼ red cabbage, shredded
Guacamole and snow pea sprouts or baby spinach, to serve

1. Cook the rice in a large saucepan of boiling water for 25 minutes or until tender. Drain and set aside to cool.

2. Meanwhile, place the baby carrots in a microwave-safe dish and microwave for 2 minutes or until tender. Place the broccolini and asparagus in a large heatproof bowl and cover with boiling water. Set aside for 2 minutes or until tender-crisp. Drain and transfer to a large bowl of iced water to cool. Drain and pat dry. Cut the asparagus and any thick stems of broccolini in half lengthways.

3. Combine the oil, lemon juice and honey in a small screw-top jar. Season. Seal and shake to combine.

4. Drizzle 2 tbs dressing over the rice. Stir to combine. Divide rice mixture among serving bowls.

5. Heat the extra 2 tsp oil in a frying pan over medium heat. Cook haloumi for 1 minute each side or until golden. Divide haloumi, carrots, broccolini, asparagus and cabbage among serving bowls. Top with guacamole and snow pea sprouts or spinach. Sprinkle with lemon rind. Drizzle with remaining dressing. Serve with lemon halves.

**COOK'S NOTE**

Always cook haloumi close to serving time, as it can become tough and rubbery as it cools.

## NUTRITION (PER SERVE)

| CALS | FAT | SAT FAT | PROTEIN | CARBS |
|------|-----|---------|---------|-------|
| 575  | 32g | 10g     | 21g     | 46g   |

● EASY   ○ FAMILY-FRIENDLY   ● GLUTEN FREE   ● LOW CAL   ○ QUICK   ○ VEGAN

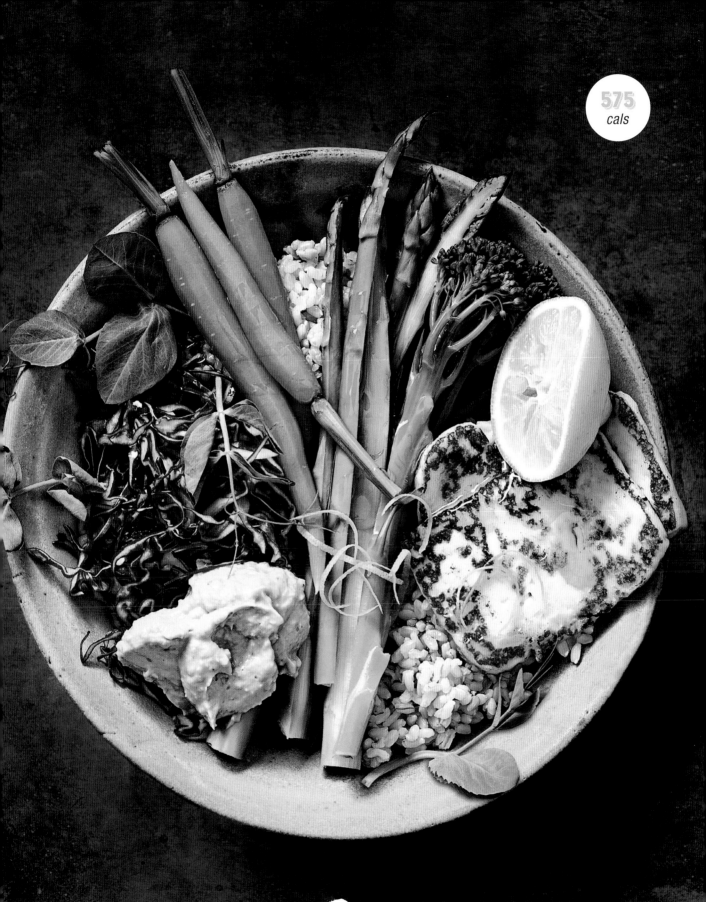

575
cals

# SPEEDY ZUCCHINI & RICOTTA PIZZA

Ready in 25 minutes, this healthier pizza uses Lebanese bread as the base and is loaded with vegies and two types of cheese. Yes, please!

**SERVES** 4  **PREP** 15 mins  **COOK** 10 mins

2 tbs extra virgin olive oil
2 garlic cloves, crushed
1 tbs finely chopped fresh
   rosemary leaves
500g light smooth ricotta
3 kale stalks
4 wholemeal Lebanese bread rounds
20g (¼ cup) finely grated parmesan
2 zucchini, very thinly sliced
200g yellow grape tomatoes, halved
¼ cup small fresh basil leaves,
   to serve

**1** Preheat oven to 220°C/200°C fan forced. Line 2 baking trays with baking paper.

**2** Combine the oil, garlic and rosemary in a bowl. Combine the ricotta and half the rosemary mixture in a separate bowl. Season.

**3** Remove and discard stems and centre veins from kale. Roughly tear leaves. Place bread on prepared trays. Spread with ricotta mixture. Sprinkle with half the parmesan. Top with the kale and zucchini. Sprinkle with the remaining parmesan. Top with the tomato, cut-side up. Drizzle with remaining rosemary mixture. Bake for 10 minutes or until vegetables soften and cheese is melted and golden. Sprinkle with basil leaves, to serve.

**COOK'S NOTE**

Have a meat eater in the family? Add chopped ham or barbecued chicken to 1-2 of these pizzas to satisfy all.

## NUTRITION (PER SERVE)

| CALS | FAT | SAT FAT | PROTEIN | CARBS |
|------|-----|---------|---------|-------|
| 462 | 20.9g | 8.5g | 22.8g | 36.3g |

★★★★★ *This pizza was quite the surprise. The ricotta made it moist and creamy. I wasn't sure about the kale, but when it was baked, it was delicious.* **SHAWNTHEPRAWN**

○ EASY   ● FAMILY-FRIENDLY   ○ GLUTEN FREE   ● LOW CAL   ● QUICK   ○ VEGAN

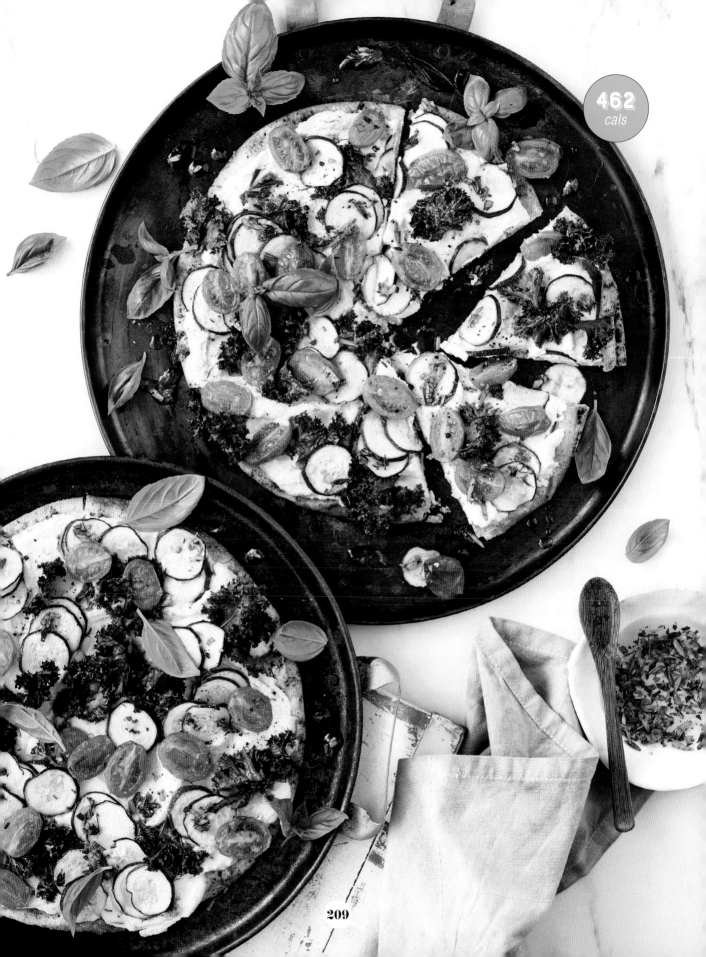

462
cals

# BRILLIANT BEETROOT

# GNOCCHI

Add colour to your dinner with this stunning dish that showcases tangy, antioxidant-rich beetroot – we've even used the leaves!

**SERVES** 4 **PREP** 15 mins **COOK** 55 mins

1 bunch small beetroot, trimmed, scrubbed, leaves reserved
45g (⅓ cup) coarsely chopped walnuts
40g butter
2 garlic cloves, crushed
2 tbs olive oil, plus extra, to serve
Balsamic vinegar, to drizzle
500g potato gnocchi
100g goat's cheese or feta, crumbled

1. Place beetroot in a saucepan and cover with water. Cover and bring to the boil over medium-high heat. Partially uncover and cook for 45 minutes or until the beetroot is tender when pierced with a skewer.

2. Meanwhile, wash and dry the beetroot leaves. Coarsely chop and set aside. Place walnut in a large frying pan. Cook, stirring, over medium heat for 3 minutes or until lightly toasted. Transfer to a plate.

3. Use a slotted spoon to transfer beetroot to a plate and set aside to cool slightly. Strain the beetroot cooking liquid into a large saucepan. Top up with boiling water from the kettle. Add a pinch of salt. Cover. Bring to the boil over medium-high heat. Add the gnocchi and cook following packet directions.

4. Meanwhile, peel beetroot and cut each into 8 wedges. Melt the butter in a frying pan over medium heat. Add the garlic. Cook, stirring, for 30 seconds or until aromatic. Add the beetroot leaves and toss until wilted. Transfer to a plate.

5. Add the oil and beetroot to the pan. Drizzle with balsamic. Season. Toss to warm through.

6. Use a slotted spoon to transfer gnocchi to the frying pan. Add leaf mixture and toss through. Divide among serving plates. Top with the goat's cheese. Drizzle with the extra oil. Sprinkle with walnut, to serve.

## NUTRITION (PER SERVE)

| CALS | FAT | SAT FAT | PROTEIN | CARBS |
|------|-----|---------|---------|-------|
| 578 | 12.2g | 12.2g | 14.8g | 39.6g |

● EASY  ● FAMILY-FRIENDLY  ○ GLUTEN FREE  ● LOW CAL  ○ QUICK  ○ VEGAN

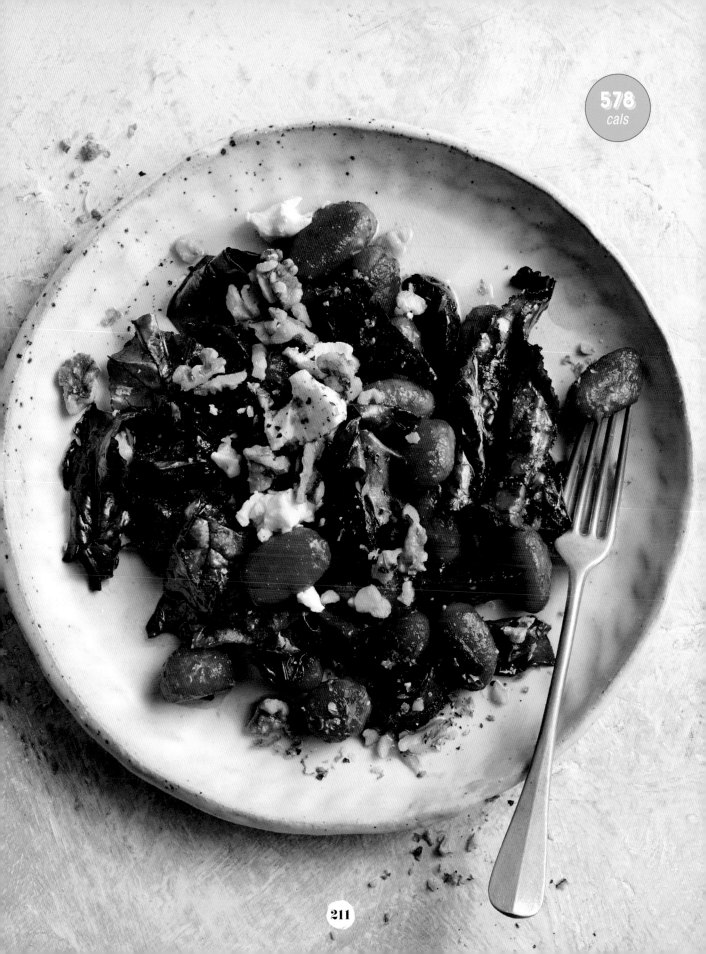

578
cals

# RISOTTO WITH
# PISELLI

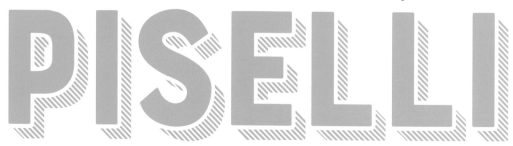

Piselli (or peas), along with cheese and white wine, are the standout flavours in this elegant northern Italian risotto that is a little on the soupy side.

**SERVES** 6  **PREP** 15 mins  **COOK** 30 mins

1L (4 cups) gluten-free vegetable stock
Pinch of saffron threads
1 tbs olive oil
1 brown onion, finely chopped
2 garlic cloves, crushed
330g (1½ cups) arborio rice
125ml (½ cup) dry white wine
150g (1 cup) frozen peas, thawed
25g (⅓ cup) finely grated parmesan
Finely grated parmesan, plus extra, to serve
20g butter, chopped

1 Place the stock and saffron in a medium saucepan over high heat. Bring just to the boil. Reduce heat to low and hold at a gentle simmer.

2 Heat the oil in a large saucepan over medium heat. Add the onion and garlic. Cook, stirring, for 5 minutes or until the onion is softened. Add the rice and cook, stirring, for 1 minute or until the grains are slightly glassy. Add the wine and cook, stirring, until the liquid is reduced by half.

3 Add a ladle, or 80ml (⅓ cup), of the stock mixture to the rice mixture and stir with a wooden spoon until liquid is absorbed. Add stock, 80ml (⅓ cup) at a time, stirring until the liquid is absorbed before adding more stock, for 20 minutes or until the rice is tender yet firm to the bite and the risotto is creamy. Add peas with the last ladle of stock.

4 Remove from the heat and stir in the parmesan. Season. Divide the risotto between serving bowls. Top with butter and extra parmesan, to serve.

**COOK'S NOTE**

A northern Italian dish, risotto can be cooked until it's thick and creamy or served slightly soupy like this delicious version.

## NUTRITION (PER SERVE)

| CALS | FAT | SAT FAT | PROTEIN | CARBS |
|------|-----|---------|---------|-------|
| 313 | 8g | 3g | 8g | 48g |

○ EASY  ● FAMILY-FRIENDLY  ● GLUTEN FREE  ● LOW CAL  ○ QUICK  ○ VEGAN

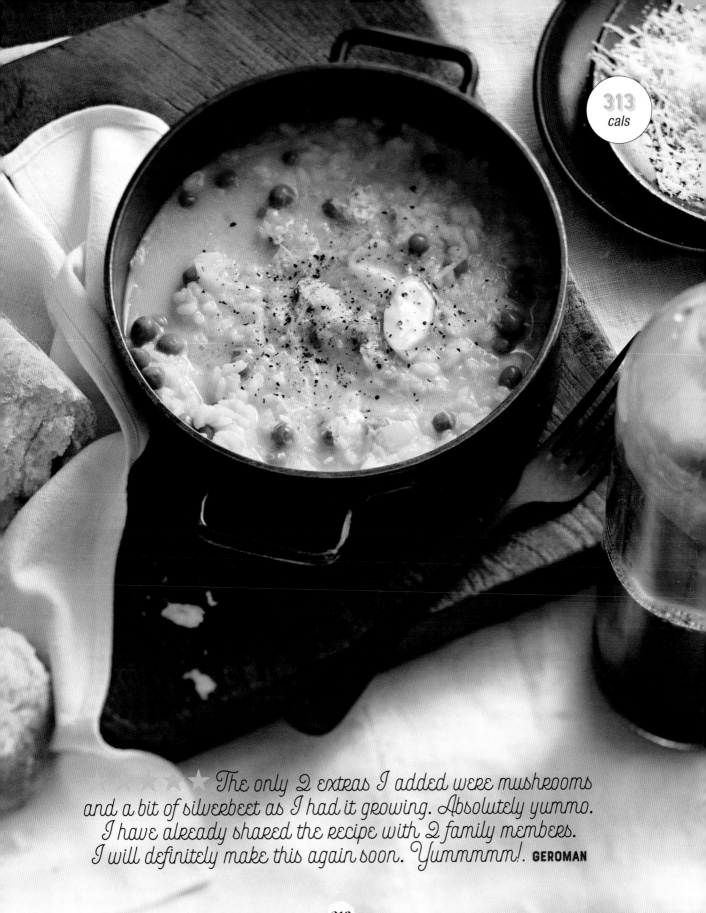

313 cals

★★★★★ The only 2 extras I added were mushrooms and a bit of silverbeet as I had it growing. Absolutely yummo. I have already shared the recipe with 2 family members. I will definitely make this again soon. Yummmm!. GEROMAN

# SNACKS

SATISFYING HUNGER-BUSTERS FOR ONE OR MORE.
THEY'RE ALL UNDER 250 CALORIES PER SERVE!

# GARLIC BREAD
# DOUGHNUTS

Cheese. Garlic bread. Yum. Make these morsels and you've hit the snack-time trifecta! The eggs and cheese will ensure you get a protein boost.

**MAKES** 20  **PREP** 25 mins (+ 1 hour 30 mins proving)  **COOK** 10 mins

80ml (⅓ cup) milk, lukewarm
2 tsp (7g sachet) dried yeast
½ tsp caster sugar
300g (2 cups) plain flour
1 tsp salt
60g butter, melted, cooled
2 eggs, lightly beaten
20g (¼ cup) finely grated parmesan
2 tbs finely chopped fresh
    continental parsley leaves
Vegetable oil, to deep-fry

**FILLING**

40g butter
4 large garlic cloves, crushed
125ml (½ cup) thickened cream
140g (1½ cups) finely grated cheddar

1 Combine the milk, yeast and sugar in a jug. Set aside for 5 minutes or until frothy. Combine the flour and salt in a large bowl. Make a well in the centre. Add the butter, egg and milk mixture. Use a wooden spoon to mix until just combined.

2 Turn dough onto a lightly floured surface and knead for 5 minutes or until smooth and elastic. Transfer to a large, lightly oiled bowl. Cover with a damp tea towel. Set aside in a warm place for 1 hour or until doubled in size.

3 Punch down dough to expel air then knead for 1-2 minutes or until smooth. Use a rolling pin to roll dough on a lightly floured surface until 7mm thick. Use a 6cm round pastry cutter to cut discs from the dough. Re-roll trimmings and continue cutting to make 20 discs in total. Place discs on a large, lightly floured tray 3cm apart. Cover lightly with a clean tea towel. Set aside for 30 minutes to prove.

4 Meanwhile, to make the filling, melt the butter in a small saucepan over low heat. Add the garlic. Cook, stirring, for 30 seconds or until aromatic. Add the cream and cheddar. Stir until melted and combined. Transfer to a bowl. Set aside to cool to room temperature.

5 Combine the parmesan and parsley in a bowl. Pour the oil into a large saucepan to come halfway up the side of the pan. Heat over medium heat until 180°C on a cook's thermometer. Cook dough discs, in batches of 4 or 5, for 1 minute each side or until puffed and deep golden. Use a slotted spoon to transfer to parmesan mixture. Press to coat. Transfer to a plate lined with paper towel. Repeat with remaining dough and parmesan mixture.

6 Spoon cooled filling into a piping bag fitted with a 7mm plain nozzle. Use a small pointed knife to pierce a hole in the side of each doughnut. Pipe some filling into each hole. Serve warm.

## NUTRITION (PER SERVE)

| CALS | FAT | SAT FAT | PROTEIN | CARBS |
| --- | --- | --- | --- | --- |
| 200 | 15.3g | 6.4g | 4.6g | 12.4g |

○ EASY  ● **FAMILY-FRIENDLY**  ○ GLUTEN FREE  ● **LOW CAL**  ○ QUICK  ○ VEGAN

200 cals

★ ★ ★ ★ ★

*Quite a few steps involved but absolutely worth it. I baked them instead of deep frying... I baked them on 220°C for 15 minutes. They come out beautifully light and tasted delicious!* **SOSUNLIGHT**

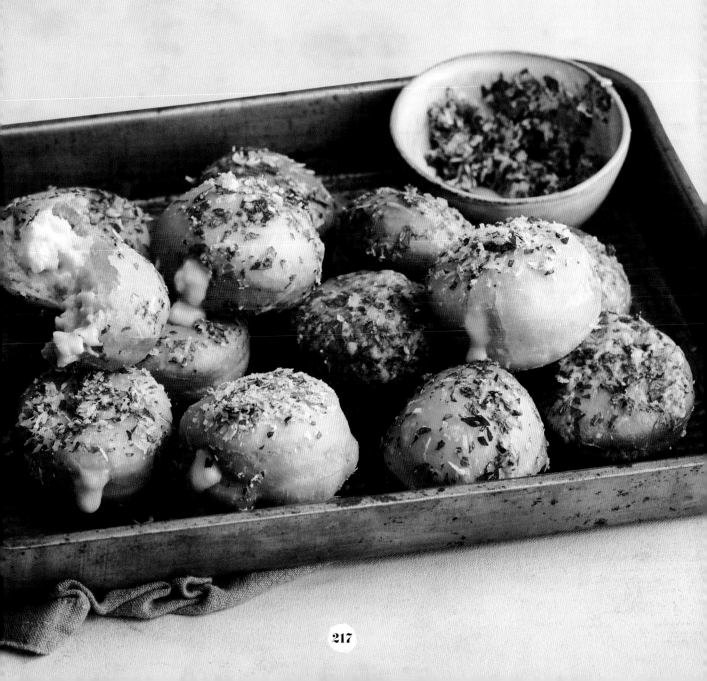

# AIR FRYER VEGIE PEEL CRISPS

Vegetable peels contain loads of nutrients, so don't toss them away – make them into crunchy salty crisps that look as amazing as they taste.

**SERVES** 4  **PREP** 10 mins  **COOK** 45 mins

Peel of 3 potatoes (see note)
Peel of 1 orange sweet potato
Peel of 1 purple sweet potato
Greek yoghurt, to serve
Sweet chilli sauce, to serve

**LEMON-HERB SALT**

1 lemon
10cm fresh rosemary sprig
30g (¼ cup) sea salt flakes

1 To make the salt, use a vegetable peeler to peel strips of rind lengthways (avoiding the pith) from the lemon. Cut each strip in half lengthways. Place the peel and rosemary in the basket of an air fryer. Cook at 70°C for 10 minutes.

2 Remove the rosemary from the air fryer. Cook peel for a further 10-15 minutes or until dry. Set aside to cool. Strip dried leaves from the rosemary sprig. Combine dried peel and rosemary leaves in a spice grinder or mortar, and grind to a powder. Add to a jar with the salt. Use the end of a wooden spoon to gently crush and combine.

3 Wash the vegetable peel and use a clean tea towel to thoroughly dry. Place in a bowl and spray lightly with olive oil. Toss to coat. Place in a single layer in the basket of the air fryer (you may need to do 2 batches). Cook at 180°C, stopping to toss once or twice, for 8-10 minutes, or until dry. Transfer to a plate. Sprinkle with the herb salt, to taste. Serve with yoghurt swirled with a little chilli sauce.

**COOK'S NOTE**

Use washed potatoes, if possible, or scrub them very well to remove all the dirt. The lemon-herb salt will keep in a sealed jar in the pantry for up to 2 months. It's delicious on top of roasted vegies.

## NUTRITION (PER SERVE)

| CALS | FAT | SAT FAT | PROTEIN | CARBS |
|------|-----|---------|---------|-------|
| 62 | 4.8g | 4.8g | 5.7g | 12.2g |

● EASY  ● FAMILY-FRIENDLY  ● GLUTEN FREE  ● LOW CAL  ○ QUICK  ○ VEGAN

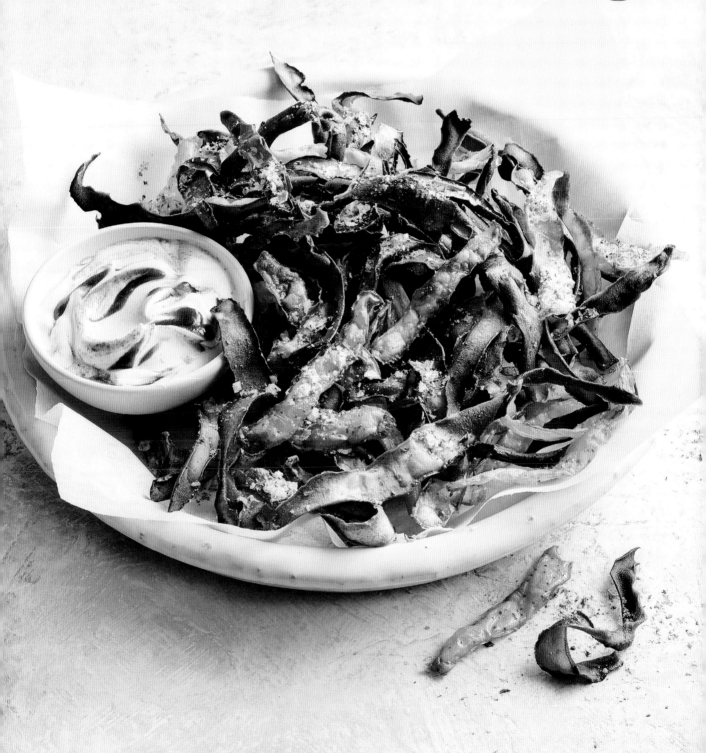

# KETO GARLIC
# BREAD

A cheesy low-carb garlic bread that's made from almond meal and covered in mozzarella – sides don't get much better than this!

**SERVES** 8  **PREP** 15 mins (+ 1 hour 10 mins standing)  **COOK** 25 mins

7g sachet instant dried yeast
1 tbs pouring cream
80ml (⅓ cup) warm water
155g (1½ cups) almond meal
2 tbs psyllium husks
1 tbs ground flaxseed
1 tsp baking powder
½ tsp salt
3 eggs, lightly beaten
60ml (¼ cup) olive oil
2 tsp apple cider vinegar
3 garlic cloves, finely chopped
100g (1 cup) grated light mozzarella
Chopped fresh continental
    parsley leaves, to serve

1. Grease a 20cm square cake pan and line with baking paper. Whisk the yeast, cream and water in a small bowl to combine. Set aside for 10 minutes or until slightly frothy.

2. Whisk the almond meal, psyllium husks, flaxseed, baking powder and salt in a large bowl. Make a well in the centre. Pour in the yeast mixture, egg, 2 tbs oil and the vinegar. Whisk well to combine. Transfer to the prepared pan. Cover loosely with plastic wrap and set aside for 1 hour or until the mixture has risen slightly.

3. Preheat oven to 200°C/180°C fan forced. Bake the bread for 15 minutes. Drizzle with remaining olive oil, and sprinkle with garlic and cheese. Bake for 10 minutes or until cheese is bubbling. Scatter with parsley, to serve.

**COOK'S NOTE**

Top the bread with halved cherry tomatoes, cut-side up, or chopped kalamata olives, after sprinkling with the cheese, if you like.

## NUTRITION (PER SERVE)

| CALS | FAT | SAT FAT | PROTEIN | CARBS |
|------|-----|---------|---------|-------|
| 232 | 24.8g | 4.4g | 8.7g | 1.3g |

★ ★ ★ ★ ★ *I'm a fairly recent convert to a keto lifestyle and have struggled with some of the bread substitutes, but this one is really tasty with a great texture. It's also really easy to make.* **CHMASON**

○ EASY   ● FAMILY-FRIENDLY   ● GLUTEN FREE   ● LOW CAL   ○ QUICK   ○ VEGAN

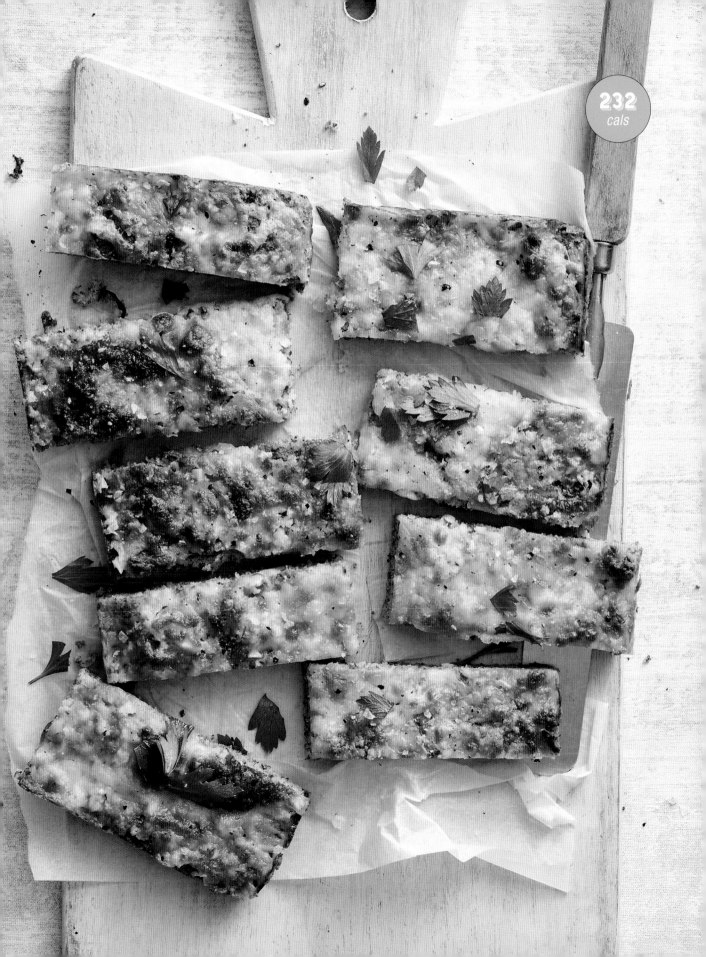

232
cals

# NICE 'N' EASY PIZZA MUFFINS

These mini pizzas are easy to make, lunch box friendly, and can be used as a base for your favourite toppings.

**MAKES** 12 **PREP** 25 mins **COOK** 20 mins

200g (1⅓ cups) plain flour, plus extra, to dust

7g sachet dry yeast

¼ tsp caster sugar

Pinch of salt

2 tbs extra virgin olive oil

160ml (⅔ cup) warm water

60ml (¼ cup) pizza sauce

140g (1¼ cups) pre-grated mozzarella

12 fresh basil leaves, plus extra, to serve

250g cherry tomatoes, halved

¼ tsp mixed herbs

**1** Preheat oven to 200ºC/180ºC fan-forced. Grease a 12-hole (⅓ cup) muffin pan.

**2** Combine the flour, yeast, sugar and salt in a large bowl. Make a well. Whisk the oil and water in a jug. Add to the well. Stir to form a soft sticky dough. Turn dough onto a lightly floured surface. Knead for 8-10 minutes or until dough springs back when lightly pressed.

**3** Roll out dough until 5mm thick. Using a 7cm round cutter, cut 12 round from the dough, re-rolling and cutting trimmings, as needed. Line the prepared muffin pan with the dough rounds, gently pushing into the holes to reach three-quarters of the way up the side of each hole.

**4** Spread the pizza sauce over the base and side of each pizza base. Sprinkle with a little mozzarella. Top with a basil leaf, then tomato. Sprinkle with remaining cheese and dried herbs. Bake for 15-20 minutes or until golden. Stand in pan for 5 minutes. Carefully transfer to a baking paper-lined wire rack to cool. Serve warm or at room temperature.

**COOK'S NOTE**

You can top these pizza bases with any of your favourite toppings, including sliced mushrooms, finely chopped capsicum and crumbled feta.

## NUTRITION (PER SERVE)

| CALS | FAT | SAT FAT | PROTEIN | CARBS |
|------|-----|---------|---------|-------|
| 151 | 6g | 2.2g | 6g | 17g |

● EASY  ● FAMILY-FRIENDLY  ○ GLUTEN FREE  ● LOW CAL  ○ QUICK  ○ VEGAN

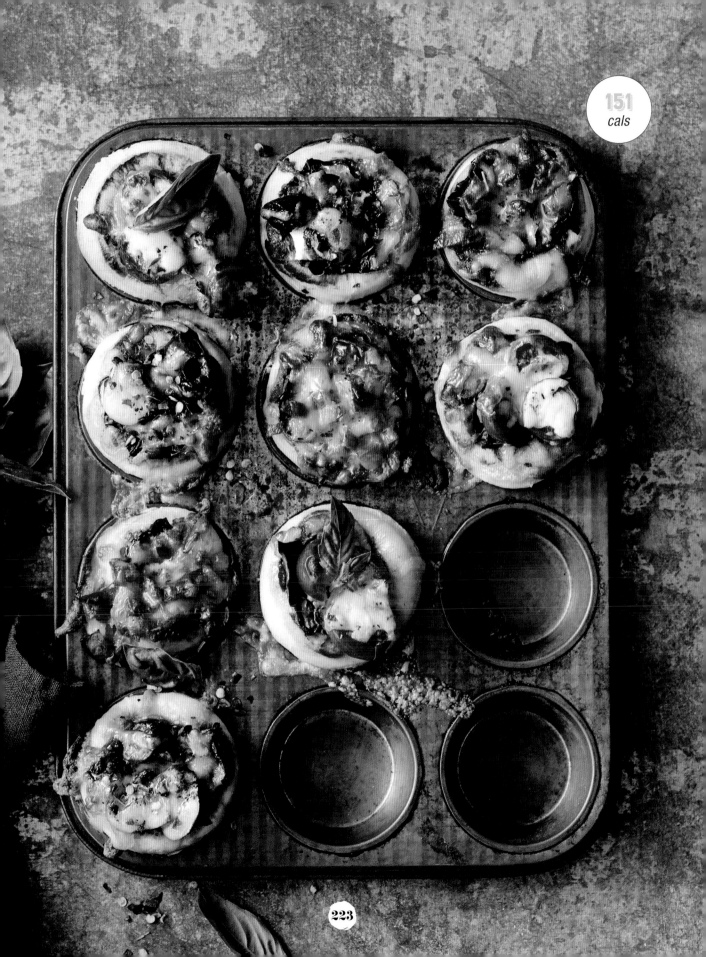

151
cals

223

# JAPANESE FRIED
# CAULIFLOWER

Coated in crispy panko breadcrumbs, these deep-fried cauliflower bites make the ideal vegetarian snack or share plate for entertaining.

**SERVES** 6  **PREP** 35 mins  **COOK** 15 mins

1 tbs light soy sauce
1 tbs cooking sake
1 tsp finely grated fresh ginger
½ cauliflower, trimmed, cut into florets
70g (1½ cups) panko breadcrumbs
50g (⅓ cup) plain flour
2 eggs
Peanut oil, to deep-fry
Tonkatsu sauce, to drizzle
Thinly sliced green shallots, Kewpie mayonnaise yuzu flavour and lemon wedges, to serve

**1** Combine the soy sauce, sake and ginger in a shallow dish. Add the cauliflower and toss to coat. Set aside, tossing occasionally, for 20 minutes to marinate.

**2** Spread the breadcrumbs on a plate and the flour on a separate plate. Crack the eggs into a shallow dish and lightly whisk to combine.

**3** Drain cauliflower, discarding the marinade. Working in batches, toss the cauliflower in the flour. Shake off excess flour. Dip in the egg to coat, then the breadcrumbs, pressing firmly to secure. Transfer to a plate.

**4** Pour enough oil into a large wok or saucepan to come one-third of the way up the side. Heat over medium-high heat to 180°C on a cook's thermometer. Working in 3 batches of about 4-5 pieces (don't overcrowd pan), deep-fry the cauliflower, turning, for 5 minutes or until golden. Use a slotted spoon to transfer to a tray lined with paper towel to drain. Repeat with remaining cauliflower.

**5** Transfer fried cauliflower to a serving dish. Season with salt. Drizzle with tonkatsu and sprinkle with shallot. Serve with mayonnaise and lemon wedges.

## COOK'S NOTE

To make it Southern fried cauliflower, ditch the tonkatsu and serve with Kewpie mayonnaise Sriracha Flavour.

## NUTRITION (PER SERVE)

| CALS | FAT | SAT FAT | PROTEIN | CARBS |
|------|------|---------|---------|-------|
| 248 | 19.3g | 3.5g | 5g | 29.7g |

○ EASY  ○ FAMILY-FRIENDLY  ○ GLUTEN FREE  ● LOW CAL  ○ QUICK  ○ VEGAN

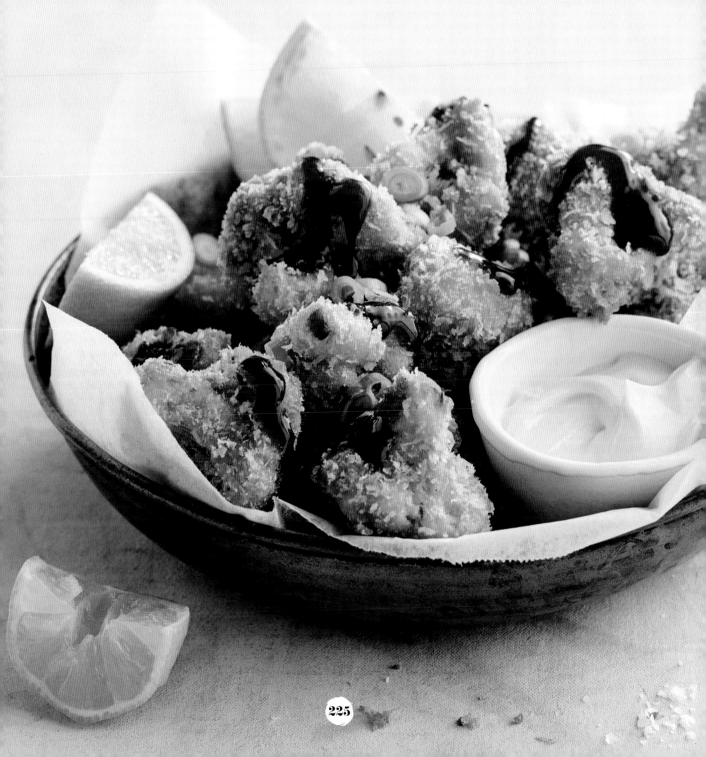

★★★★★
*Loved this, great vegetarian change from fried chicken.
Kids didn't even realise it was cauliflower – they devoured it.* **BLYMER**

# ZUCCHINI & FETA
# MUFFINS

These easy zucchini muffins are made with ricotta and reduced-fat feta so they're still super-cheesy but are much better for you.

**MAKES** 12 **PREP** 20 mins (+ cooling) **COOK** 40 mins

2 tbs extra virgin olive oil
3 green shallots, trimmed,
   thinly sliced
1 garlic clove, crushed
1 tsp finely grated lemon rind
2 zucchini, trimmed
320g (2 cups) wholemeal
   self-raising flour
Pinch of cayenne pepper
375ml (1½ cups) buttermilk
125g (½ cup) low-fat fresh ricotta
2 eggs
125g reduced-fat feta, crumbled

**1** Preheat oven to 190°C/170°C fan forced. Lightly grease twelve 80ml (⅓ cup) muffin pan holes.

**2** Combine the oil, shallot and garlic in a small frying pan over a low heat. Cook until the oil just starts to bubble and the shallot has softened slightly. Transfer to a small bowl (with all the oil). Stir in the lemon rind and set aside to cool.

**3** Use a julienne peeler to cut the zucchini into long thin strips, or coarsely grate.

**4** Place the flour in a large bowl. Add the cayenne pepper and season with salt. Make a well in the centre. Whisk the buttermilk, ricotta and eggs in a jug until smooth. Pour into the well with the shallot mixture and stir until just combined. Fold in nearly all the zucchini and feta, reserving a little of both to decorate the muffin tops.

**5** Divide mixture among the prepared muffin holes (they will be very full) and top with the reserved zucchini and feta. Bake for 30-35 minutes or until the muffins spring back when gently touched. Set aside for 5 minutes to cool slightly. Use a flat-bladed knife to gently loosen each muffin and remove from the pans. Eat warm or at room temperature.

**COOK'S NOTE**

Cooled muffins can be frozen. Wrap individually in foil, then place in airtight sealable bags and freeze for up to 1 month.

## NUTRITION (PER SERVE)

| CALS | FAT | SAT FAT | PROTEIN | CARBS |
|------|-----|---------|---------|-------|
| 176 | 6.8g | 2.3g | 8.7g | 18g |

● EASY  ● FAMILY-FRIENDLY  ○ GLUTEN FREE  ● LOW CAL  ○ QUICK  ○ VEGAN

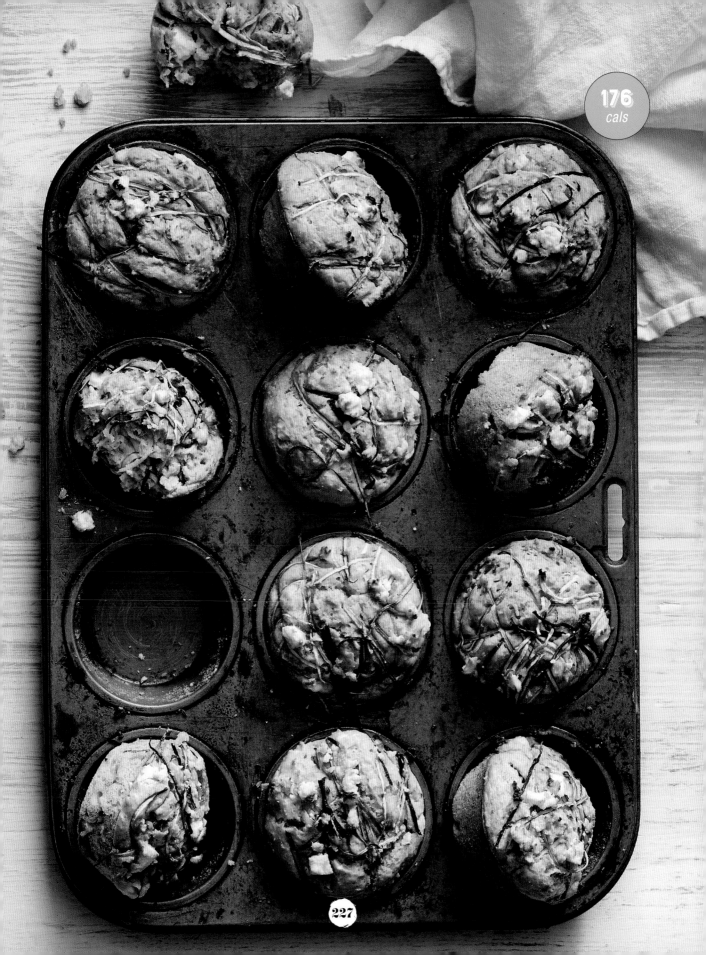

# VEGETABLE PEEL & FETA LOAF

Packed with flavour, this feta, vegie and herb loaf is a tasty way to use up carrot, sweet potato and potato peel. Every slice is nice!

**SERVES** 8 **PREP** 20 mins **COOK** 45 mins

225g (1½ cups) self-raising flour
1 tsp baking powder
3 eggs
125ml (½ cup) milk
2 tsp sea salt flakes
200g (2 cups) vegetable peelings (such as carrot, sweet potato and potato), coarsely chopped (see note)
1 cup chopped fresh continental parsley leaves and stems, plus extra leaves (optional), to serve
4 green shallots, finely chopped
1 tbs fresh thyme leaves, finely chopped
150g feta, chopped

1 Preheat oven to 180°C/160°C fan forced. Grease the base and sides of a 11 x 21cm loaf pan and line with baking paper.

2 Sift the flour and baking powder into a large bowl. Add the eggs, milk and salt. Stir to combine.

3 Add the vegie peel, parsley, shallot and thyme. Mix until just combined. Gently fold in the feta. Spoon mixture into the prepared pan. Bake for 40-45 minutes or until a skewer inserted into the centre comes out clean. Top the loaf with extra parsley, if using. Serve warm or at room temperature.

**COOK'S NOTE**

Wash and scrub the vegies before peeling to remove any unwanted dirt.

## NUTRITION (PER SERVE)

| CALS | FAT | SAT FAT | PROTEIN | CARBS |
|------|-----|---------|---------|-------|
| 205 | 6.7g | 3.5g | 9.7g | 24.9g |

★★★★★

*I often get the munchies mid morning, so this is a good snack to have on hand. One slice is all I need to feel satisfied.* **CSHORE**

● EASY  ○ FAMILY-FRIENDLY  ○ GLUTEN FREE  ● LOW CAL  ○ QUICK  ○ VEGAN

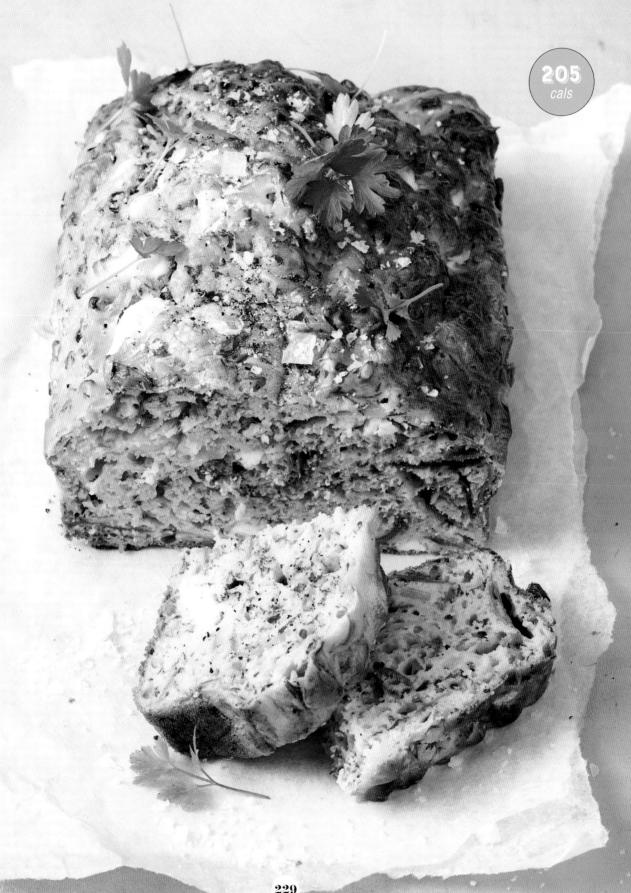

205
cals

# CHEESY VEGETARIAN 'SAUSAGE' ROLLS

Made from sweet potato, lentils and mushrooms, these easy vego sausage rolls will have even the meat eaters reaching for another one.

**MAKES** 16  **PREP** 10 mins (+ 15 mins cooling)  **COOK** 40 mins

1 tbs olive oil
1 brown onion, finely chopped
2 garlic cloves
2 tsp Vegemite
Pinch dried chilli flakes (optional)
200g button mushrooms, coarsely chopped
125g (1 cup) grated sweet potato
400g can brown lentils, rinsed, drained
2 tsp fresh thyme leaves
150g colby cheese, cut into 1cm pieces
2 sheets frozen puff pastry, just thawed
1 egg, lightly whisked
Tomato relish or tomato sauce, to serve

1 Preheat oven to 200°C/180°C fan forced. Line 2 baking trays with baking paper.

2 Heat the oil in a large frying pan over medium heat. Add the onion. Cook, stirring often, for 4-5 minutes or until softened. Add the garlic, Vegemite and chilli (if using). Cook, stirring, for 30 seconds or until aromatic. Add the mushroom and cook, stirring often, for 5 minutes or until softened and the liquid is evaporated. Add the sweet potato and cook, stirring, for 2 minutes or until softened. Stir in the lentils and thyme. Season. Transfer to a large heatproof bowl. Set aside, stirring often, for 15 minutes or until cool. Stir in the cheese.

3 Cut each pastry sheet in half. Place one-quarter of the sweet potato mixture in a log shape along 1 long edge of the pastry. Brush the opposite edge with egg. Roll up tightly to enclose. Repeat with remaining pastry halves and filling. Cut each roll into 4 equal pieces and place, seam-side down, on the prepared trays.

4 Brush pastry with egg and use a sharp knife to score lines crossways across the tops of each roll. Bake for 25 minutes or until golden. Serve with tomato relish or sauce.

**COOK'S NOTE**

Replace the sweet potato with grated pumpkin or use a mixture of vegies such as zucchini, carrot and peas, if you like.

## NUTRITION (PER ROLL)

| CALS | FAT | SAT FAT | PROTEIN | CARBS |
|------|-----|---------|---------|-------|
| 178 | 10g | 5.5g | 6.5g | 14.1g |

○ EASY  ● **FAMILY-FRIENDLY**  ○ GLUTEN FREE  ● **LOW CAL**  ○ QUICK  ○ VEGAN

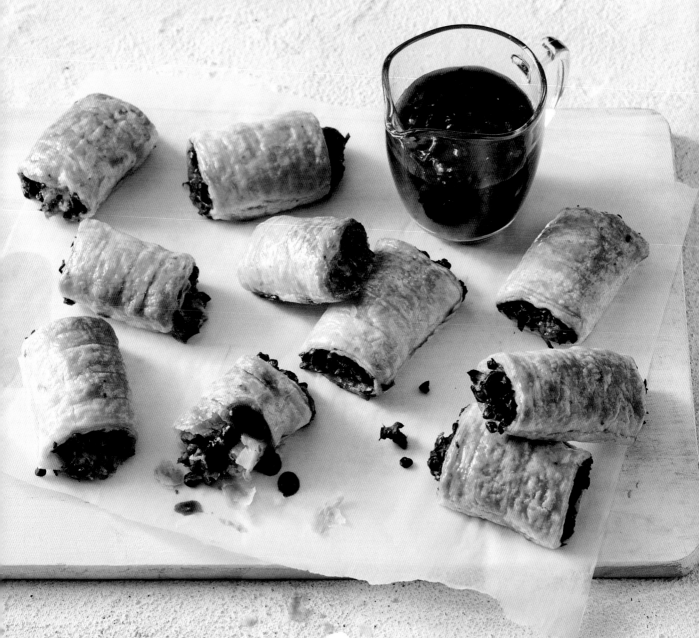

179 cals

★ ★ ★ ★ ★

*These are yum, that big a hit with the family they want them made again so they can take to school for lunches.* **FPV141**

# SPICED CAULI & HUMMUS DIP

Get your entertaining into full swing with this loaded hummus dip. It looks pretty on the table and the flavours are amazing. Prepare for it to go fast!

**SERVES** 12  **PREP** 15 mins  **COOK** 15 mins

2 tbs extra virgin olive oil, plus extra, to serve
500g cauliflower, cut into small florets
1 tsp ground cumin
1 tsp smoked paprika
30g (¼ cup) walnut halves
1 cup fresh continental parsley leaves, coarsely chopped
¼ cup fresh mint leaves, coarsely chopped
¼ small red onion, finely chopped
1 tsp finely grated lemon rind, plus lemon wedges, to serve
200g tub roasted beetroot hummus
500g hummus
50g (½ cup) lightly salted roasted chickpeas
Warmed Turkish bread, sliced, to serve

**1** Heat the oil in a large frying pan over medium-high heat. Cook cauliflower, tossing occasionally, for 8-10 minutes or until golden and tender. Add cumin and paprika. Toss to coat. Cook, tossing, for 1 minute or until aromatic. Season. Remove from pan and drain on paper towel.

**2** Return pan to the heat. Add walnuts. Cook, tossing, for 2 minutes or until toasted. Transfer to a board and coarsely chop. Set aside. Combine the parsley, mint, onion and lemon rind in a bowl.

**3** Spread beetroot hummus over a serving platter. Top with plain hummus, spreading to slightly cover. Sprinkle half the herb mixture over hummus. Top with cauliflower, then remaining herb mixture. Sprinkle with walnut and chickpeas. Drizzle with extra oil. Serve with lemon wedges and bread.

**COOK'S NOTE**

For a lighter and less filling option, serve with pita crisps rather than Turkish bread.

## NUTRITION (PER SERVE)

| CALS | FAT | SAT FAT | PROTEIN | CARBS |
|------|------|---------|---------|-------|
| 245 | 18.7g | 2.1g | 6.5g | 9.9g |

★★★★★

*Easy, fast and healthy!* **LAGUDA76**

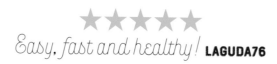

● EASY  ○ FAMILY-FRIENDLY  ○ GLUTEN FREE  ● LOW CAL  ● QUICK  ○ VEGAN

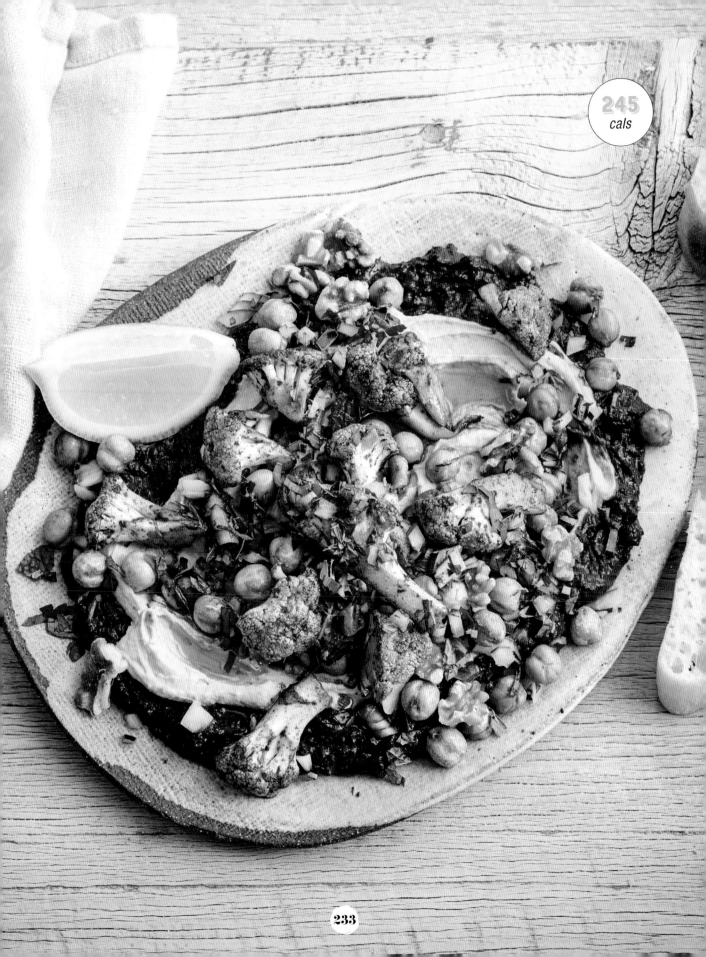

# ROAST PUMPKIN & RICOTTA
# MUFFINS

These healthy little muffins are a great lunch box filler or light snack for you or the kids. Make a batch on the weekend and you're sorted for the week.

**MAKES** 9  **PREP** 20 mins  **COOK** 45 mins

500g pumpkin, peeled, cut into 1cm pieces
1 large red onion, cut into thin wedges
1 tbs chopped fresh rosemary leaves
310g (2 cups) wholemeal spelt flour
3 tsp baking powder
2 eggs
2 tbs extra virgin olive oil
125ml (½ cup) unsweetened almond milk
125g (½ cup) fresh ricotta, plus extra 60g (¼ cup)
75g baby spinach, coarsely chopped
Toasted pepitas, to serve

1 Preheat oven to 190°C/170°C fan forced. Line a large baking tray with baking paper. Place pumpkin and onion on prepared tray. Sprinkle with rosemary and lightly spray with olive oil. Bake for 25 minutes or until pumpkin is tender.

2 Line nine 185ml (¾ cup) muffin pans with paper cases. Sift the flour and baking powder into a large bowl. Whisk the eggs, oil, milk and ricotta in a jug. Add to the flour mixture and stir until just combined. Stir through the roasted vegetables and spinach.

3 Divide mixture among prepared muffin pans. Top with extra ricotta. Bake for 20-22 minutes or until muffins are golden and a skewer inserted into the centres comes out clean. Sprinkle with pepitas, to serve.

**COOK'S NOTE**

Use regular wholemeal plain flour in place of the spelt flour, if you prefer, and cow's milk instead of almond milk, if that is what you have on hand.

## NUTRITION (PER SERVE)

| CALS | FAT | SAT FAT | PROTEIN | CARBS |
|------|-----|---------|---------|-------|
| 239  | 9g  | 2.7g    | 9g      | 28.3g |

★★★★★

*The kids are always hungry after school, so I've been baking lots of these as a healthy snack before dinner. They devour them!* **SHAWNTHEPRAWN**

○ EASY   ● FAMILY-FRIENDLY   ○ GLUTEN FREE   ● LOW CAL   ○ QUICK   ○ VEGAN

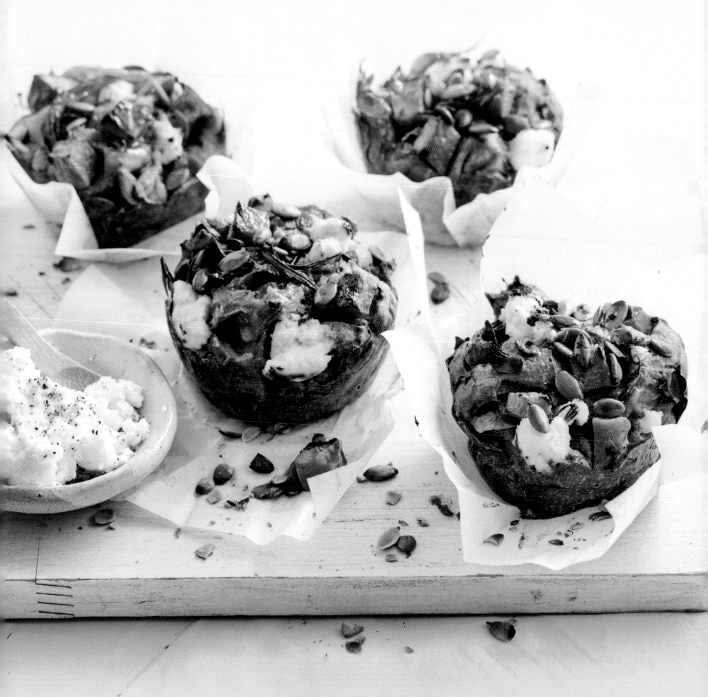

# CHEESY KETO
## SNACKS

Keto snacks don't get much better than these quick and easy cheesy crackers. Served with smashed avo, they'll be the hit of the party.

**SERVES** 8 **PREP** 10 mins **COOK** 15 mins

155g (1½ cups) pre-grated 3-cheese blend
80g (⅔ cup) almond meal
60g cream cheese
1 egg, lightly beaten
1 tsp finely chopped fresh rosemary leaves
1 tbs sunflower seeds
2 tsp linseeds
Smashed avocado, to serve

1 Preheat oven to 180°C/160°C fan forced. Line 2 baking trays with baking paper. Place the grated cheese, almond meal, cream cheese and 60ml (¼ cup) water in a medium saucepan. Cook, stirring with a wooden spoon, over medium heat for 3 minutes or until melted and combined. Remove from the heat.

2 Working quickly, add the egg and rosemary to the pan and beat until well combined. Divide mixture between prepared trays. Scatter with sunflower seeds and linseeds. Cover each tray with a sheet of baking paper. Use a rolling pin to roll each mixture to a thin 2-3mm-thick rectangle.

3 Remove the baking paper. Use a pizza cutter or sharp knife to cut each rectangle into wedges.

4 Bake for 12 minutes or until golden. Set aside to cool. Serve with a bowl of smashed avocado for dipping.

**COOK'S NOTE**

These snacks will store for up to 2 days in an airtight container at room temperature.

## NUTRITION (PER SERVE)

| CALS | FAT | SAT FAT | PROTEIN | CARBS |
|------|------|---------|---------|-------|
| 205 | 18.1g | 6.8g | 9.1g | 0.6g |

★★★★★ *Made this today and the whole family loved it. Kids especially.* **GLAMORENTERTAINMENTAUSTRALIA**

● EASY  ● FAMILY-FRIENDLY  ● GLUTEN FREE  ● LOW CAL  ● QUICK  ○ VEGAN

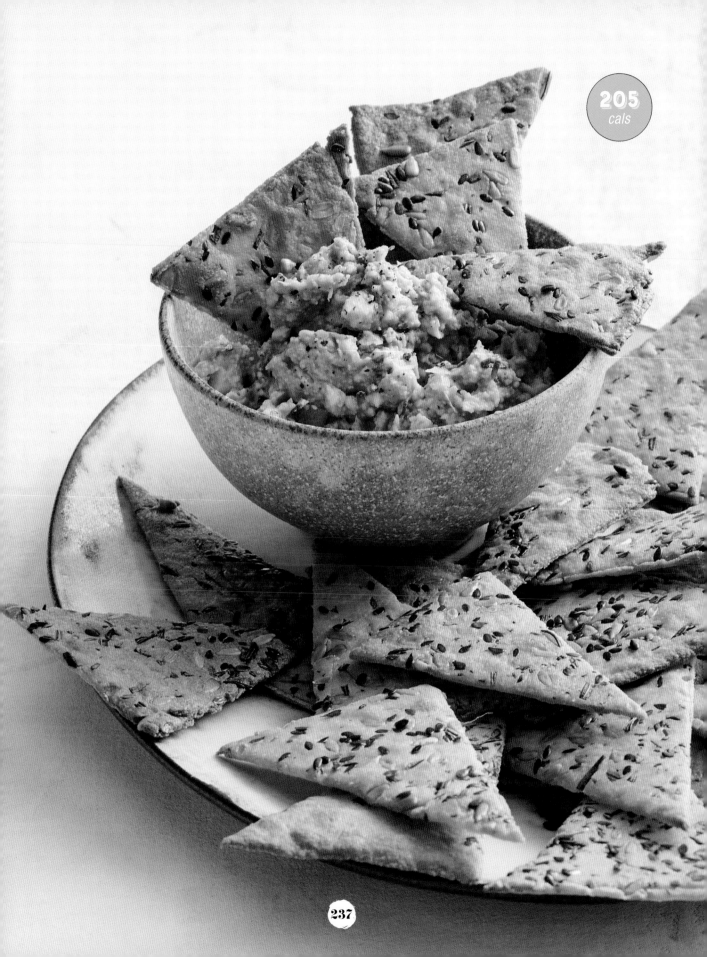

205
cals

237

# CHEESY CAULIFLOWER MUFFINS

Make a big batch of these vegie-packed muffins – they're a brilliant hunger buster. Plus, they're low-fat and low-cal to boot!

**MAKES** 9 **PREP** 20 mins **COOK** 35 mins

400g cauliflower, cut into florets
235g (1½ cups) wholemeal spelt flour
3 tsp baking powder
3 eggs
2 tbs extra virgin olive oil
1 carrot, peeled, coarsely grated
1 zucchini, coarsely grated
40g (½ cup) finely grated parmesan, plus extra 20g (¼ cup)
6 green shallots, thinly sliced

1 Preheat oven to 190°C/170°C fan forced. Line nine 185ml (¾ cup) muffin pans with paper cases. Process 350g cauliflower in a food processor until it resembles coarse crumbs. Place in a heatproof bowl, cover and microwave for 3 minutes. Drain.

2 Add the remaining cauliflower florets to the cauli crumbs. Cover. Microwave for 3 minutes. Drain. Reserve 9 small florets.

3 Sift the flour and baking powder into a large bowl. Whisk the eggs and oil in a jug. Add to the flour mixture and stir until just combined. Stir through the cauli crumb mix, carrot, zucchini, parmesan and half the shallot.

4 Divide mixture among prepared muffin pans. Place 1 reserved cauliflower floret on top of each and gently press partway into the mixture. Bake for 20-25 minutes or until muffins are golden. Combine remaining shallot and extra parmesan. Sprinkle over the muffins, to serve.

**COOK'S NOTE**

Serve muffins warm with mixed salad leaves and dressing for a light lunch, or serve alone as a filling afternoon snack.

## NUTRITION (PER SERVE)

| CALS | FAT | SAT FAT | PROTEIN | CARBS |
|------|-----|---------|---------|-------|
| 191 | 8.1g | 2.3g | 9.1g | 19.8g |

● EASY   ● FAMILY-FRIENDLY   ○ GLUTEN FREE   ● LOW CAL   ○ QUICK   ○ VEGAN

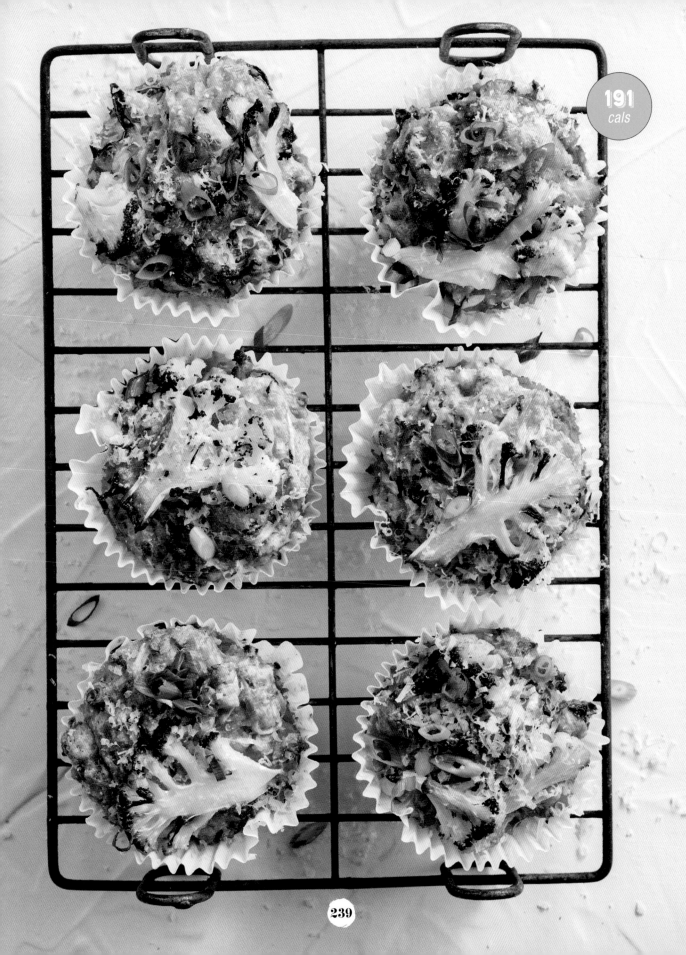

191
cals

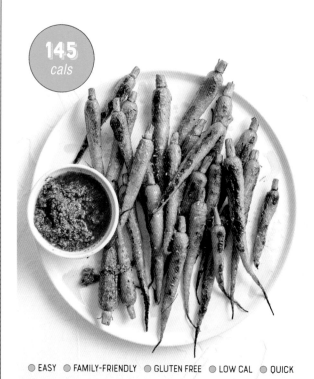

**145** *cals*

# CARROT TOP
# PESTO

**SERVES** 4 **PREP** 10 mins

**1** Place **1½ tbs toasted pepitas**, **1 garlic clove** and **1 small dried red chilli** in a small food processor. Pulse until coarsely chopped.

**2** Add **1 cup chopped washed and dried carrot tops** and **125ml (½ cup) olive oil** to the food processor. Pulse until mixture is well combined.

**3** Transfer both mixtures to a bowl. Stir in **25g (⅓ cup) finely grated parmesan** and **an extra 1 tbs olive oil**. Serve with **roasted baby carrots** for dipping.

## NUTRITION (PER SERVE)

| CALS | FAT | SAT FAT | PROTEIN | CARBS |
|------|-----|---------|---------|-------|
| 145  | 6.6g | 2g     | 8.3g    | 11.1g |

● EASY  ● FAMILY-FRIENDLY  ● GLUTEN FREE  ● LOW CAL  ● QUICK

**228** *cals*

# SALSA FUN
# AVOCADO

**SERVES** 2 **PREP** 15 mins

**1** Cut **1 avocado** in half and remove the stone. Combine **1 large finely chopped ripe tomato**, **2 tsp finely chopped red onion**, **1 tbs each of chopped fresh coriander leaves** and **fresh lime juice**, and **1 tsp extra virgin olive oil** in a small bowl.

**2** Season. Place **3-4 tbs Greek-style yoghurt** in the cavity of each avo half. Top with the tomato salsa and some corn chips. Sprinkle with **ground paprika** and serve.

## NUTRITION (PER SERVE)

| CALS | FAT | SAT FAT | PROTEIN | CARBS |
|------|-----|---------|---------|-------|
| 228  | 17.9g | 5.1g  | 5.3g    | 7.1g  |

● EASY  ● FAMILY-FRIENDLY  ● GLUTEN FREE  ● LOW CAL  ● QUICK

# APPLE BRUSCHETTA
## SLICES

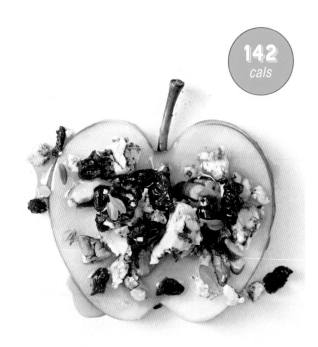

**142** cals

**MAKES** 6 **PREP** 10 mins

1. Use a mandoline to thinly slice **1 red apple** lengthways into heart-shaped pieces. Keep the stem on the middle slice attached, if possible. Remove any seeds. Place the slices on a serving platter.

2. Top with **50g crumbled creamy blue cheese**, some **toasted chopped pecans** for crunch, and **finely chopped dried cranberries** and **lemon thyme** for a pop of colour. Drizzle with **maple syrup,** to serve.

## NUTRITION (PER 2 SLICES)

| CALS | FAT | SAT FAT | PROTEIN | CARBS |
|------|-----|---------|---------|-------|
| 142 | 8.8g | 3.6g | 4g | 2g |

● EASY ● FAMILY-FRIENDLY ● GLUTEN FREE ● LOW CAL ● QUICK

# RAINBOW VEG BEETROOT
## DIP

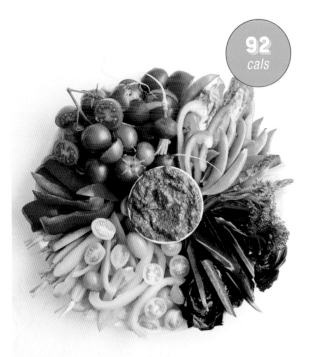

**92** cals

**SERVES** 8 **PREP** 15 mins

1. Drain a **450g can baby beetroot** and coarsely chop. Place beetroot, **2 tbs fresh lemon juice** and **1 tsp each of ground cumin and coriander** in a bowl. Season.

2. Use a stick blender to blend until smooth and thickened. Stir in **½ cup Greek-style yoghurt**. Transfer dip to a serving bowl on a serving platter. Arrange sliced vegetables in rainbow colours around the bowl. Serve.

## NUTRITION (PER SERVE)

| CALS | FAT | SAT FAT | PROTEIN | CARBS |
|------|-----|---------|---------|-------|
| 92 | 4.8g | 2.9g | 2.5g | 7.5g |

● EASY ● FAMILY-FRIENDLY ● GLUTEN FREE ● LOW CAL ● QUICK

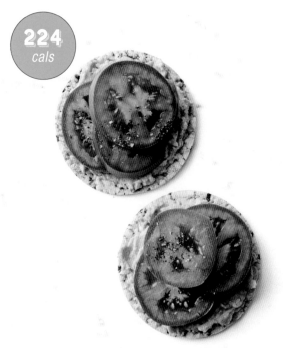

**224** cals

# AVO & TOMATO CORN
# THINS

**SERVES** 1 **PREP** 5 mins

1 Place **2 multigrain corn thins** on a small serving plate. Spread each with **2 tsp mashed avocado**.

2 Slice **1 roma tomato** crossways. Arrange slices on top of the avocado. Season and serve.

## NUTRITION (EACH)

| CALS | FAT | SAT FAT | PROTEIN | CARBS |
|------|-----|---------|---------|-------|
| 224 | 4.7g | 1.2g | 2g | 12.7g |

● EASY  ● FAMILY-FRIENDLY  ● GLUTEN FREE  ● LOW CAL  ● QUICK

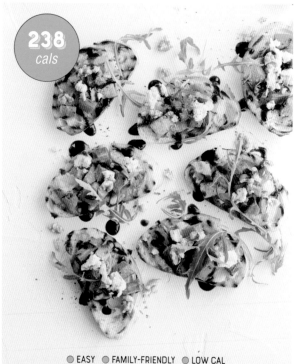

**238** cals

# ROAST VEGIE
# TOASTIES

**SERVES** 8 **PREP** 10 mins **COOK** 30 mins

1 Preheat oven to 200°C/180°C fan forced. Line 2 baking trays with baking paper. Place **4 cups chopped mixed vegetables (such as pumpkin, sweet potato and carrot)**, **1 garlic bulb, cloves separated**, and **2 tsp chopped herbs (such as rosemary, thyme or sage)** on prepared trays. Drizzle over **2 tbs extra virgin olive oil**. Season. Toss. Roast for 30 minutes or until the vegetables are golden and tender.

2 Grill or toast **8 slices sourdough bread**. Squeeze garlic out of skins into a bowl. Mash. Spread thinly over toast. Top with the vegies. Sprinkle with **50g each of blue cheese and feta**, crumbled, **baby rocket** and **½ cup nuts, toasted, chopped (such as walnuts, almonds or pine nuts)**. Drizzle with **1 tbs balsamic glaze** to serve.

## NUTRITION (EACH)

| CALS | FAT | SAT FAT | PROTEIN | CARBS |
|------|-----|---------|---------|-------|
| 238 | 11.4g | 2.7g | 8.8g | 23.3g |

● EASY  ● FAMILY-FRIENDLY  ● LOW CAL

# BROCCOLI QUINOA
# NUGGETS

**SERVES** 6 **PREP** 15 mins **COOK** 20 mins

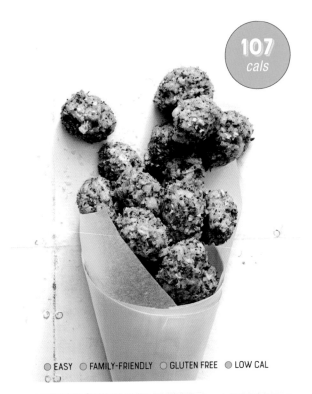

**107** cals

1 Preheat oven to 200°C/180°C fan forced. Line a large baking tray with baking paper.

2 Blanch **200g broccoli florets**. Drain and refresh under cold water. Squeeze out excess water. Place in a food processor and process until coarsely chopped. Add **½ cup quinoa flakes**, **½ cup cooked quinoa**, **60g grated haloumi**, **2 chopped green shallots** and **2 lightly beaten eggs**. Pulse to combine. Season.

3 Shape level tablespoonfuls firmly into oval shapes and place on prepared tray. Spray with oil. Bake for 15 minutes or until golden. Serve hot.

## NUTRITION (EACH)

| CALS | FAT | SAT FAT | PROTEIN | CARBS |
|------|-----|---------|---------|-------|
| 107 | 4.1g | 1.6g | 7.6g | 2.3g |

○ EASY  ○ FAMILY-FRIENDLY  ○ GLUTEN FREE  ● LOW CAL

# POACHED EGG & KALE
# SNACK

**SERVES** 2 **PREP** 5 mins **COOK** 5 mins

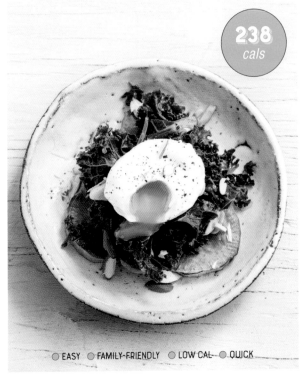

**238** cals

1 Spray a large non-stick frying pan with oil and heat over medium-high heat. Add **1 crushed garlic clove**. Cook, stirring, for 30 seconds or until aromatic. Add **100g trimmed kale, washed and chopped**. Cook, stirring, for 2-3 minutes or until wilted.

2 Arrange **2 poached eggs**, wilted kale and **½ small avocado, sliced**, on **2 slices toasted wholegrain bread**. Sprinkle with **baby herbs, if desired**. Season with **pepper**, to serve.

## NUTRITION (PER SERVE)

| CALS | FAT | SAT FAT | PROTEIN | CARBS |
|------|-----|---------|---------|-------|
| 238 | 14g | 4g | 11g | 14g |

○ EASY  ○ FAMILY-FRIENDLY  ○ LOW CAL  ○ QUICK

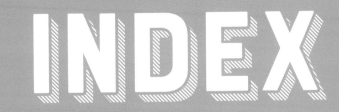

# INDEX

ALL OF YOUR FAVOURITE DISHES BY ALPHABETICAL
ORDER, KEY GUIDE, MAIN INGREDIENT AND MEAL TYPE.

# The Eat Real Diet
# ALPHABETICAL INDEX

Looking for a favourite recipe? Here's a list of every recipe in this book to make it easier to find the ones you want to cook again and again.

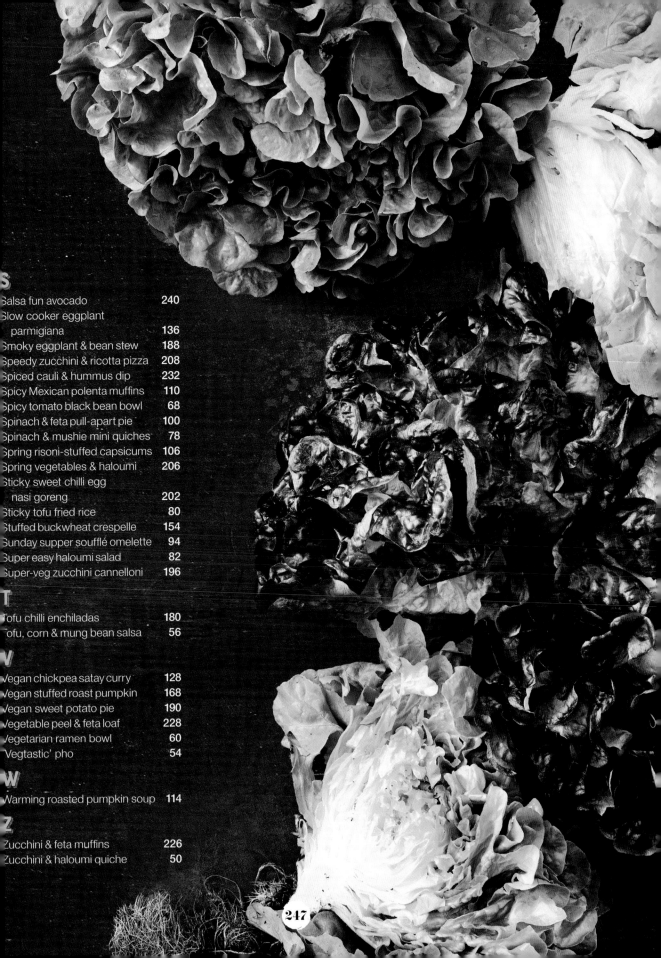

# The Eat Real Diet
# INDEX BY KEY GUIDE

Every dish in this book is low-cal for everyday eating whether a light meal, main or snack. Here, you can easily find gluten-free or vegan dishes, and more.

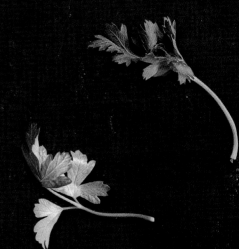

# The Eat Real Diet

# INDEX BY MAIN INGREDIENT

Check out this list of star ingredients to find your main protein
or vegie preference – it will make shopping and cooking easier.

# The Eat Real Diet
# INDEX BY MEAL TYPE

Keep track of your daily calorie intake with our light meal and main meal options, then fill in the gaps with our satisfying low-cal snacks.

## LIGHT MEALS
### (LESS THAN 400 CALORIES)

| | |
|---|---|
| Asparagus filo frittatas | 92 |
| 'Bacon' & sweet potato spaghetti | 108 |
| Beetroot vegie burgers | 72 |
| Cauli rice & korma tofu | 84 |
| Choc, fruit & oat brekky bowl | 42 |
| Creamy tomato soup with ravioli | 76 |
| Crispiest sweetcorn fritters | 38 |
| Curried tofu & vegetable patties | 88 |
| Eggplant, feta & quinoa salad | 112 |
| Flaky lentil & silverbeet pies | 96 |
| Healthy banana waffles | 40 |
| Healthy leek & broccoli soup | 48 |
| Healthy Mexican fried rice | 90 |
| Healthy potato-crust quiche | 104 |
| Japanese stuffed sweet potatoes | 116 |
| Jatz cracker & spinach quiche | 86 |
| Keto pancakes | 32 |
| Lemony turmeric & lentil soup | 102 |
| Lentil, brussels & mushie medley | 58 |
| Loaded chickpea pancakes | 120 |
| Mexican zucchini slice | 70 |
| Miso roasted eggplant | 64 |
| Muffin pan frittatas | 74 |
| One-pan sweet potato & egg hash | 44 |
| One-pot keto zucchini alfredo | 62 |
| Overnight chia porridge | 34 |
| Pumpkin & basil risotto | 46 |
| Pumpkin crustless quiche | 98 |
| Pumpkin curry with tofu | 52 |
| Punchy protein breakfast bowl | 36 |
| Quick Thai tofu noodle salad | 66 |
| Red cabbage with pumpkin falafel | 118 |
| Spicy Mexican polenta muffins | 110 |
| Spicy tomato black bean bowl | 68 |
| Spinach & feta pull-apart pie | 100 |
| Spinach & mushie mini quiches | 78 |
| Spring risoni-stuffed capsicums | 106 |
| Sticky tofu fried rice | 80 |
| Sunday supper soufflé omelette | 94 |
| Super easy haloumi salad | 82 |
| Tofu, corn & mung bean salsa | 56 |
| Vegetarian ramen bowl | 60 |
| 'Vegtastic' pho | 54 |
| Warming roasted pumpkin soup | 114 |
| Zucchini & haloumi quiche. | 50 |

## MAIN MEALS
### (LESS THAN 600 CALORIES)

| | |
|---|---|
| Bean & beets mushroom burgers | 170 |
| Black bean & chipotle soup | 186 |
| Brilliant beetroot gnocchi | 210 |
| Caprese lasagne roll-ups | 200 |
| Cauliflower parmigiana tray bake | 184 |
| Cheesy pumpkin & potato bake | 176 |
| Cheesy stuffed cauliflower | 132 |
| Clean-out-the-fridge risotto | 182 |
| Crispy caesar salad | 164 |
| Curried lentil & vegetable pie | 194 |
| Dhal-stuffed sweet potatoes | 174 |
| Easy falafel tray bake | 204 |
| Eggplant parmigiana lasagne | 162 |
| Fast falafel & black rice tabouli | 160 |
| 5-ingredient ravioli lasagne | 172 |
| Healthy Tuscan bread soup | 138 |
| Indian-style 'butter' broccoli | 166 |
| Japanese tofu katsu | 156 |
| Lasagne with zucchini lattice | 142 |
| Mediterranean vegetable Wellington | 140 |
| Mexican burrito lasagne | 178 |
| Mexican mushroom tacos | 198 |
| Mexican taco pizzas | 130 |
| Mushroom & lentil lasagne | 124 |
| Mushroom stroganoff pasta bake | 150 |
| North Indian paneer curry | 152 |
| One-pan vegetable biryani | 134 |
| Pumpkin & kale lazy lasagne | 192 |
| Pumpkin diane | 158 |
| Quick super-green mee goreng | 148 |
| Quick vegetarian minestrone | 126 |
| Quick vegetarian pad Thai | 144 |
| Risotto primavera | 146 |
| Risotto with piselli | 212 |
| Slow cooker eggplant parmigiana | 13 |
| Smoky eggplant & bean stew | 188 |
| Speedy zucchini & ricotta pizza | 208 |
| Spring vegetables & haloumi | 206 |
| Sticky sweet chilli egg nasi goreng | 202 |
| Stuffed buckwheat crespelle | 154 |
| Super-veg zucchini cannelloni | 196 |
| Tofu chilli enchiladas | 180 |
| Vegan chickpea satay curry | 128 |
| Vegan stuffed roast pumpkin | 168 |
| Vegan sweet potato pie | 190 |

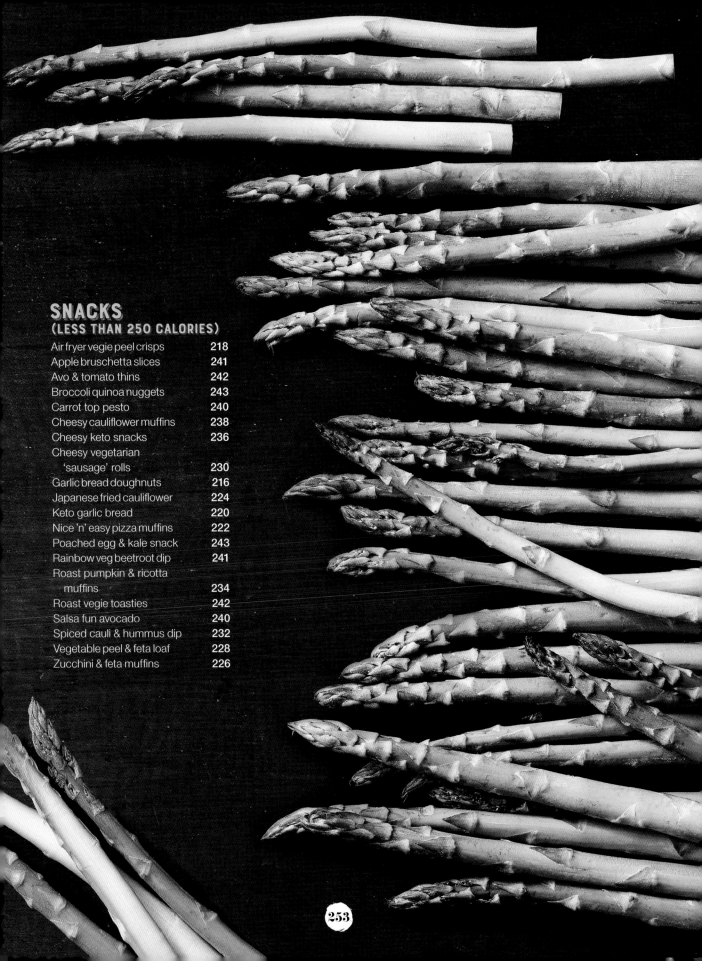

## SNACKS
### (LESS THAN 250 CALORIES)

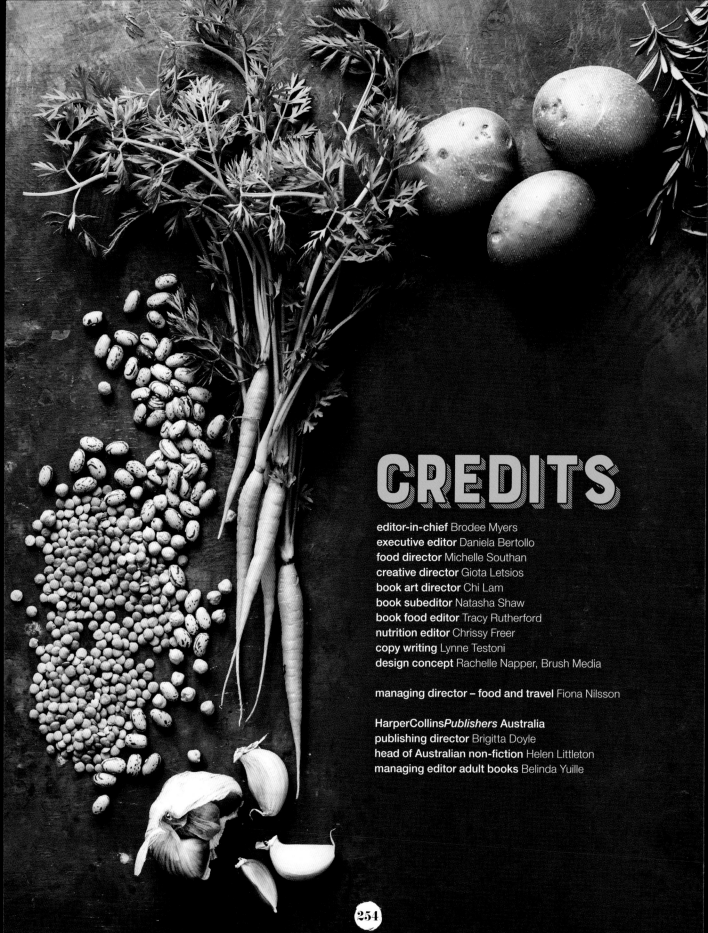

# CREDITS

**editor-in-chief** Brodee Myers
**executive editor** Daniela Bertollo
**food director** Michelle Southan
**creative director** Giota Letsios
**book art director** Chi Lam
**book subeditor** Natasha Shaw
**book food editor** Tracy Rutherford
**nutrition editor** Chrissy Freer
**copy writing** Lynne Testoni
**design concept** Rachelle Napper, Brush Media

**managing director – food and travel** Fiona Nilsson

**HarperCollins*Publishers* Australia**
**publishing director** Brigitta Doyle
**head of Australian non-fiction** Helen Littleton
**managing editor adult books** Belinda Yuille

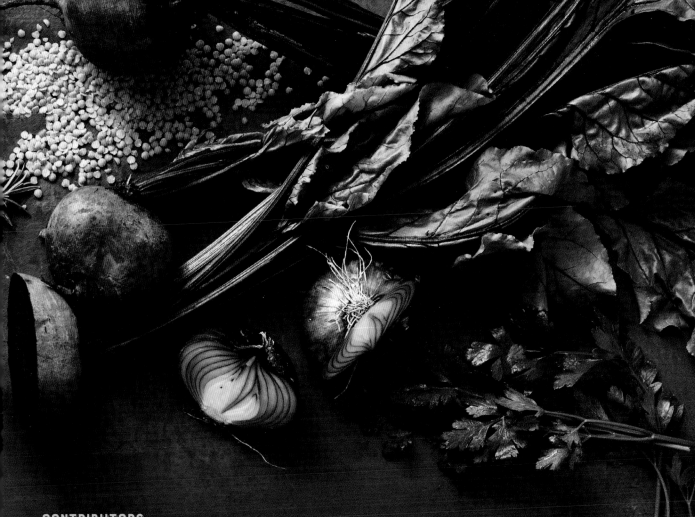

## CONTRIBUTORS

### Recipes

Alison Adams, Charlotte Binns-Mcdonald, Claire Brookman,
Lucy Busuttil, Amber de Florio, Chrissy Freer, Amira Georgy,
Cathie Lonnie, Liz Macri, Kate Murdoch, Lucy Nunes,
Tiffany Page, Miranda Payne, Kerrie Ray, Tracy Rutherford,
Michelle Southan, Katrina Woodman

### Photography

Guy Bailey, Chris L. Jones, Vanessa Levis, Andy Lewis,
Sam McAdam-Cooper, Jeremy Simons, Brett Stevens,
Craig Wall, Andrew Young

**HarperCollins*Publishers***

Australia • Brazil • Canada • France • Germany • Holland
• Hungary • India • Italy • Japan • Mexico • New Zealand
• Poland • Spain • Sweden • Switzerland • United Kingdom
• United States of America

First published in Australia in 2022
by HarperCollins*Publishers* Australia Pty Limited
ABN 36 009 913 517
harpercollins.com.au

A catalogue record for this book is available
from the National Library of Australia.

ISBN 978 1 4607 6047 5

Colour reproduction by Splitting Image Colour Studio,
Clayton, Victoria, Australia

Printed and bound in China by RR Donnelley

8 7 6 5 4 3 2   22 23 24 25 26

# THANK YOU

At taste.com.au HQ, we're super proud of the delicious and fuss-free healthy meals that make up Eat Real. *The Eat Real Diet* is a cookbook for our times, giving you access to more than 100 low-calorie recipes to create amazing light meals, mains and snacks, and increase your daily vegetable intake. We'd like to thank everyone on the Taste team who contributed to this book – from our foodies to photographers, stylists, designers, subeditors and the digital team. Each recipe is a result of amazing passion and teamwork.

A huge thank you as well to Brigitta Doyle and Helen Littleton, our partners at HarperCollins. We're very thankful for your expertise and support.

We'd also like to thank ... you, the audience of taste.com.au! Thousands of passionate cooks visit our site every day to plan, cook and share their reviews, ratings and recipe twists and tips. We love hearing about your passion for cooking and the gusto with which you make our recipes, so keep those reviews, comments and photos coming. And continue to eat real!

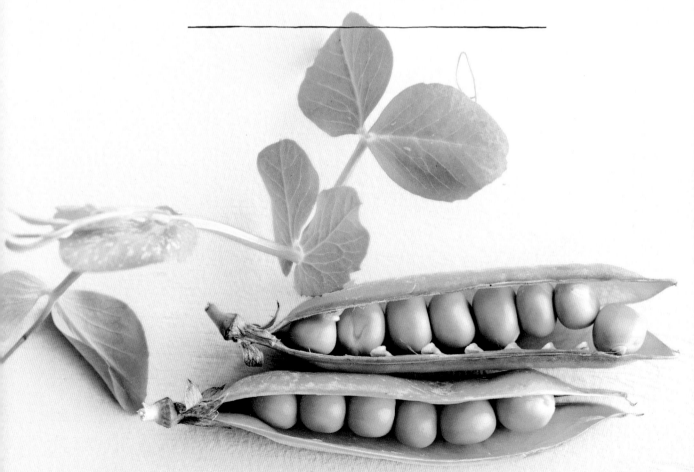